COMMUNITY–ACADEMIC PARTNERSHIPS FOR EARLY CHILDHOOD HEALTH

T0136914

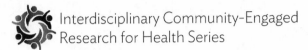 Interdisciplinary Community-Engaged
Research for Health Series

The *Interdisciplinary Community-Engaged Research for Health* series aims to bridge the gap between researchers and practitioners to facilitate the development of collaborative, equitable research and action. The reality of persistent health disparities and structural inequalities highlights the need for new strategies that are social justice-driven. Traditionally, efforts have tended to be institution-based, "expert"-focused, and silo-specific. To promote health equity, diverse stakeholders with different types of expertise need to work together to solve real-world problems. This series publishes books that recognize the importance of diverse collaboration and equip readers from a variety of backgrounds with the tools and vision to center community voice in research for action.

Series Editors:

Farrah Jacquez
University of Cincinnati

Lina Svedin
University of Utah

Advisory Board:

Sherrie Flynt Wallington
George Washington University

Jennifer Malat
University of Cincinnati

Kristin Kalsem
University of Cincinnati

Kathleen Thiede Call
University of Minnesota

Andriana Abariotes
University of Minnesota

COMMUNITY–ACADEMIC PARTNERSHIPS FOR EARLY CHILDHOOD HEALTH

Interdisciplinary Community-Engaged Research for Health Series

Volume 1

Edited by Farrah Jacquez & Lina Svedin

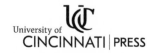

University of CINCINNATI | PRESS

About the University of Cincinnati Press

The University of Cincinnati Press is committed to publishing rigorous, peer-reviewed, leading scholarship accessibly to stimulate dialog among the academy, public intellectuals, and lay practitioners. The Press endeavors to erase disciplinary boundaries in order to cast fresh light on common problems in our global community. Building on the university's long-standing tradition of social responsibility to the citizens of Cincinnati, state of Ohio, and the world, the Press publishes books on topics that expose and resolve disparities at every level of society and have local, national, and global impact.

University of Cincinnati Press, Cincinnati 45221
Copyright © 2021

Published in 2020

ISBN (hardback) 978-1-947602-68-7
ISBN (e-book, PDF) 978-1-947602-69-4
ISBN (e-book, EPUB) 978-1-947602-70-0

Jacquez, Farrah Mariél, editor. | Svedin, Lina M., editor.
Community-academic partnerships for early childhood health / edited
  by Farrah Jacquez and Lina Svedin.
Other titles: Interdisciplinary community engaged research for health ; v. 1. Description:
Cincinnati: University of Cincinnati Press, 2019. | Series:
  Interdisciplinary community engaged research for health; volume 1 |
  Includes bibliographical references and index.
Identifiers: LCCN 2019021666 | ISBN 9781947602687 (hardback) | ISBN
  9781947602694 (epub) | ISBN 9781947602700 (pdf)
Subjects: MESH: Child Health | Community-Based Participatory
  Research – methods | Infant Health | United States
Classification: LCC RJ61 | NLM WS 440 | DDC 618.92--dc23
LC record available at https://lccn.loc.gov/2019021666

Designed and produced for UC Press by Jennifer Flint
Typeset in Granjon LT Std
Printed in the United States of America
First Printing

Contents

1 Community-Engaged Research to Improve Health
  and Well-Being for Young Children   1
  Farrah Jacquez, Lina Svedin

2 Enhancing the Arkansas Birthing Project through Technology   21
  Sarah Rhoads, Zenobia Harris, Hari Eswaran

3 A Place-Based Approach to Early Childhood Wellness in
  Cincinnati: Communities Acting for Kids Empowerment (CAKE) 35
  Michael Topmiller, Farrah Jacquez, Jamie-Lee Morris

4 Finding Our Way as a Cross-Systems Team: Lessons Learned
  from an Interdisciplinary Research Team   57
  Karen Ruprecht, Angela Tomlin, Shoshanna Spector

5 Improving Racial Equity in Birth Outcomes:
  A Community-Based, Culturally Centered Approach   83
  Katy Kozhimannil, Rachel Hardeman, Rebecca Polston

6 Creating Transformational Nonprofit/University Partnerships
  in Public Health: Lessons Derived from Collaboration between
  Room to Grow and Columbia University   111
  *Allyson Crawford, Bethany C. Brichta, Ruby L. Engel, Joanna
  Groccia, Anna E. Holt, Tonya Pavlenko, Karen Juliet Sanchez,
  Christopher Wimer*

7 Building Strong Partnerships with the Puerto Rico WIC Program
  for Promoting Healthy Lifestyles in Early Childhood
  and a Long-Lasting Culture of Health   147
  Maribel Campos, Cristina Palacios, Alexandra Reyes

8 In Search of Child Welfare and Child Health Collaboration   167
   Lina Svedin, Tonya Myrup, Kristine Campbell

9 Interdisciplinary Community-Engaged Research (ICER)
   for Health: Growing in Understanding and Effectiveness   193
   Lina Svedin, Farrah Jacquez

Bios   217

Index   225

Community–Academic Partnerships for Early Childhood Health

Chapter 1

Community-Engaged Research
to Improve Health and Well-Being
for Young Children

Farrah Jacquez
University of Cincinnati

Lina Svedin
University of Utah

Interdisciplinary Community-Engaged Research for Health is a series that aims to bridge the gaps between science and practice and between different disciplines to facilitate collaborative research toward improved health and health equity. In each volume, authors will describe the specific tools they have used (both successfully and unsuccessfully) to work together and the impact of those efforts on health outcomes. Taken together, the *Interdisciplinary Community-Engaged Research for Health* series will provide a road map for inclusive interdisciplinary collaborations toward specific goals. Volume 1 describes research collaborations focused broadly on improved outcomes but more specifically on increased equity in early childhood health.

The authors included in this volume are researchers and community members who were part of the first cohort of the Robert Wood Johnson Foundation's Interdisciplinary Research Leaders (IRL) program. The IRL program funds three-person teams, composed of two researchers and one community member, using the power of applied research to engage the community to define and explore a question, and then applies findings in real time to create measurable changes. The following chapters describe the process IRL teams used to work together to improve the health of young children.

To increase the potential for research to lead to real-world action and systems-level change, the IRL program requires collaboration between academic and community partners. Similarly this volume has purposely been designed to reach a wide audience of academics, community leaders, practitioners, and students who are interested in collaborating to do applied research. Although the editors of this volume are both researchers, each chapter describes collaborations between diverse teams of researchers and community members working for early childhood health promotion across the United States. As researchers, we have chosen this path because we care deeply about the health and well-being of the communities we work with and the outcomes at stake. We have met people from all over the country who share these passions and have stories to tell from their own journeys. Whether you are a community organizer or an agency leader, a student or faculty member, a researcher or a policy analyst, an elected official or a system-change agent, this book is for you. To help you follow the threads that weave the subsequent chapters together, this introductory chapter presents the rationale for this volume and some of the main ideas and concepts that support the research presented in the subsequent chapters. We aim to inspire and encourage excellence in research that respects the inherent knowledge and wisdom of communities and is conducted with community benefit as the ultimate goal. We share our teams' research processes and experiences of conducting community-engaged research in hopes that you will someday, in the not too distant future, feel empowered and equipped to do the same.

Setting Our Sights to Change the Course

We are not alone in our passion for community-engaged health research. Persistent health inequities resulting from structural inequality have motivated many researchers and research-funding institutions to seek new ways to move the needle toward social equity across a number of sectors. Traditionally, health promotion and intervention efforts tend to be institution-based, "expert"-driven, and silo-specific. To achieve health equity, diverse stakeholders with different types of knowledge and expertise need to work together to solve real-world problems. Scientists and faculty members from different disciplines and research orientations need to integrate their skills for translational outcomes. Researchers need to work collaboratively with community partners, not just "grasstops," such as directors of agencies and presidents of organizations, but also community members who are feeling the real-world effects of health inequities. Without the expertise of those who are experiencing structural inequality, any efforts to overcome health inequities will have limited potential for change.

Collaborating across disciplines and through scientist/practitioner lines sounds ideal, but in reality the challenges can derail even the most well-intentioned efforts. The vocabulary used by community residents, nonprofit agencies, and researchers from different disciplines can all vary dramatically from one another. The goals and value systems held by different stakeholders can lead to entirely different perspectives on problems and their possible solutions. In order to work together toward health equity, there is a need not only to recognize the importance of collaboration but also to have the tools and vision to understand how to carry it out.

Scholars from various disciplines wanting to pursue community-engaged research currently have few high-quality sources to turn to for methodological advice and best practices. Considerable and important work resulting from community-academic partnerships is currently being published, expanding our understanding of the potential impact of community-engaged research. The methodological coverage of the process of this work, however, is scant at best. Journal articles publishing results from studies claiming to be community-engaged research frequently make summary statements such as "we engaged the community all throughout this process." Not only does this leave much to the imagination in terms of being able to verify how and to what extent "the community" was involved, it insinuates that community-engaged research looks just like traditional research but with extra people. We hope that by illuminating the process we will arm future researchers with the tools needed to plan, conduct, and advocate for this work. For example, most of the chapters in this volume emphasize the need to be flexible through significant changes in personnel, political landscape, and/or policies. Similarly, authors describe the amount of time it took to get through the process as being longer than anticipated. These perspectives can prepare future researchers to invest more time and energy into the maintenance of collaborative relationships and build flexibility in research plans.

By providing a structured discussion of the nuts-and-bolts processes needed to conduct funded, team-based, community-engaged research in the United States, this volume shares perspectives that increase our ability to refine and make community-engaged research more effective and transparent. While the chapters reflect on unique research questions and projects, each chapter describes what the community partnership looked like, how it was created, and how it influenced and shaped the research questions. Furthermore, we highlight the process of investigation, what worked well, and where the teams of researchers encountered successes and challenges. The chapters present research questions and objectives that address a larger effort to promote the health of young children in the United States, and in doing so shed light on the scalable, replicable processes and methods of community-engaged research.

The authors represented in the volume were selected to do this community-engaged research on a competitive grant application basis and represent a unique team-based research approach. Research partners represent top teaching and research institutions in the United States, and community partners represent nonprofit organizations, state and local agencies, state and regional community organizations, and for-profit community service organizations. The breadth of experience and expertise that the volume communicates is unique and can serve as the foundation for a much-needed methodological development conversation as well as insight into excellence in research that truly utilizes the strengths of both researcher and practitioner in team-based science.

Community-Engaged Research: Definitions and Prevalence

As a scholar-practitioner community, we consider community-engaged research valuable and feasible, and, in terms of health, it may be our best chance at promoting and supporting lasting societal change. However, interdisciplinary community-engaged research (ICER) comes with many challenges. While some of these barriers and challenges have prevented scholars from engaging in ICER, we set out to showcase how teams of researchers and community members have worked to overcome them. We encourage others to conduct this type of research and to promote high-quality, strengths-based research that respects community culture.

Our definition of community-engaged research refers to collaborations between researchers and community members for the "mutually beneficial exchange of knowledge and resources in a context of partnership and reciprocity" (Driscoll 2008). The primary goals of community-engaged research are action, impact, and community benefit; a secondary goal is the dissemination of the research results to the academic community to contribute knowledge toward future research, interventions, and policy development. Although community-engaged research exists across almost all disciplines, the words used to describe it vary widely. Educators and social scientists are more likely to describe community-engaged work as *action research* or *participatory action research*. Within higher education, scholars often use the terms *civic engagement* or *community-engaged scholarship*. Health systems researchers tend to discuss *consumer engagement*. Public health and academic medicine most often use the term *community-based participatory research* (CBPR) to describe research conducted in partnership with community members to improve healthcare and health outcomes.

The common theme among all disciplines is matching the knowledge and methodology expertise of researchers with the local expertise and lived experiences of community members to collaborate for change. Scholars have described community-academic partnerships on a continuum ranging from cooperation to coordination to collaboration to partnership, with each step indicating more equity in decision-making (Winer and Ray 2000). Community and academic partners should decide together where on the continuum they want their work to be, based on their research question and their specific goals. Although any point on the continuum falls under the umbrella of community-engaged research, there is increasing recognition of the benefits of shared leadership between community and academic partners. The National Institutes of Health have described the amplified impact, flow, and communication that comes with enhancing collaboration on all steps of the research process (CTSA 2011). Specifically, they posit that shared leadership increases the potential for broader benefits in health outcomes, larger community impact, and stronger bidirectional trust built as a foundation for future collaboration.

Although community-engaged research is prevalent across disciplines targeting diverse outcomes, work in the health arena, in particular, has grown exponentially in the last decade. Recent recommendations from international organizations emphasize the necessary role of community participation in improving population health and reaching health equity (WHO Regional Office 2012; WHO 2016). Research-funding mechanisms appear to be following their lead and requiring community-engaged research in grant proposals. The National Institutes of Health's Clinical and Translational Science Award (CTSA) program supports a national network of medical research institutions that work together to improve the translational research process to get more treatments to more patients more quickly. In 2017 fifty-seven medical institutions across the United States collectively received half a billion dollars in CTSA funding. CTSA funding has historically required that institutions include a community-engagement component in their program's activities, resulting in a major incentive for researchers to do community-engaged research and a major need for effective community collaborations. The Patient-Centered Outcomes Research Institute (PCORI) is a nonprofit, nongovernmental organization that was authorized by Congress in 2010 to "improve the quality and relevance of evidence available to help patients, caregivers, clinicians, employers, insurers, and policymakers make better-informed health decisions" (PCORI 2018). Since 2017 PCORI has funded $1.6 billion in research aimed directly at responding to patients' circumstances and preferences by meaningfully involving patients in the research process.

Increased funding has led to considerable growth in the amount of community-engaged research happening across the United States and internationally, which has led to an increased need for academic outlets disseminating this type of work. Over the past ten years several journals have been developed with the specific mission to disseminate community-engaged work. Perhaps most prominently, the Community-Campus Partnerships for Health has been publishing *Progress in Community Health Partnerships*, often described as the journal of CBPR, since 2007. Estalished in 2008, *Clinical and Translational Science* is a medical journal highlighting original research, bridging laboratory discoveries with the diagnosis and treatment of human disease. Two newer journals provide specific opportunities for authors to describe the process of working with communities in research: *Gateways: International Journal of Community Research and Engagement* and *Collaborations: A Journal of Community-Based Research and Practice*. The number of articles featuring community-engaged research has also increased exponentially within traditional, well-established journals. Several prominent journals that regularly feature community-engaged work are *Social Science and Medicine*, *Health Promotion Practice*, the *Journal of Healthcare for the Poor and Underserved*, the *American Journal of Public Health*, *Ethnicity and Disease*, the *Journal of Cancer Education*, and the *Journal of Urban Health*.

Why Community-Engaged Research?

The environmental scientists Carolina Balzacs and Rachel Morello-Frosch have described the ways that community-based participatory research (or research that includes shared leadership between community and academic partners) can improve the relevance, rigor, and reach of scientific research (Balzacs and Morello-Frosch 2013). First, shared decision-making between community members and scientists ensures that research is asking the right questions, thereby making research more relevant in the real world. Individuals who are experiencing poor health or are historically on the receiving end of health inequities can provide the perspective of relevance to lived experiences, while scientists can provide perspective of the relevance in relation to existing scientific research.

Second, collaborating with community members improves the rigor of scientific research by promoting the validity of study design, improving data collection, and ensuring that data interpretation is in line with real-world experience. Measurement validity will be higher when individuals who are similar to participants help choose tools. Participant recruitment can improve dramatically when community members are doing the asking, particularly in marginalized populations, where mistrust of scientists runs high. Understanding the meaning and implications of results always reflect the bias of the scientist conducting the research; including community members in the interpretation process ensures that the interpretation is understood in the context of lived experiences.

Third, shared leadership ensures a wide reach of dissemination, increasing not only the contribution to the scientific literature but also the potential for change in regulatory and policy arenas. Taken together, the rigor-relevance-reach framework helps to conceptualize how community-engaged research can provide better research evidence to promote a culture of health and to move the needle toward eliminating health inequities.

In response to the recent boom in community-engaged research in health fields, scholars have attempted to provide definitive evidence that collaborating with community partners can improve health

outcomes. Despite considerable interest and requests from a wide
spectrum of health-related sectors, comprehensive meta-analyses of
community-engaged research processes and outcomes have proven to
be difficult. Most challenging—the disparate vocabulary researchers
use to describe research along the community-engagement continuum
makes synthesizing the literature extremely challenging (Rifkin 2014;
Sarrami-Foroushani et al. 2014). Several suggestions for conceptualizing
community engagement to improve comparability have emerged in the
last decade, including subcategorizations of community participation
(South et al. 2017), organization by key concepts of community participation (Sarrami-Foroushani et al. 2014), and the use of "community-
academic partnerships" as the "single conceptual definition to unite
multiple research disciplines and strengthen the field" (Drahota et al.
2016, 163). Community participation is better thought of as a process
rather than a research method because any participation is going to
be context-specific and therefore difficult to generalize across studies
(Rifkin 2014).

Despite the challenges, several reviews of the literature have established associations between community-engaged research and improved
health outcomes, particularly among marginalized populations. One
systematic review and meta-analysis of 319 community-engaged public
health research studies found that community-engaged interventions are
effective in improving health behaviors, health outcomes, self-efficacy,
and social support (O'Mara-Eves et al. 2013). The authors analyzed the
data for systematic methodological biases and found that the benefits to
health outcomes appear to be robust. Another systematic review of the
role of community-engaged research in health promotion among disadvantaged populations found that 88 percent of reviewed interventions
improved health outcomes and 60 percent reduced health inequities

(Cyril et al. 2015). In their review of sixty-four studies of community participation in health systems research, George et al. (2015) found that most of the existing literature detailed improvements in service availability, accessibility, and acceptability when partnering with communities. In a study of two hundred CBPR projects, researchers found that not only community involvement in research but also the quality of community-academic partnerships were associated with immediate and distal health outcomes (Oetzel et al. 2018).

Community-Engaged Research and Improving Health in the United States

The research presented in this volume is built on the notion that research can and should inform policy change and that policy change in and of itself is important for improving health—but that it is not enough. Our community partners and years of conducting research that has not had enough impact, and on-the-ground benefit, have convinced us that research needs to be less top-down, better informed by listening to the people it studies, and responsive to how the community views and prioritizes those needs. We see the need to include and engage researchers and community members as equal partners, with a stake in the questions asked and the outcomes studied, in order to create significant change. By conducting research that engages the communities we study in a meaningful way, we can help create and sustain community change to support health, and by engaging in this community-engaged research, we see a potential for deep and lasting societal change with regard to health.

In an effort to create and support cultures of health in US communities, the teams featured in this volume focus on early childhood and health. Developments and challenges in this area have the potential to impact the health of individuals in the short term and long term. The challenges that the research teams look into—early childhood and health—are felt across the United States. In this sense, the research conducted and presented in this volume has a bearing on conditions and communities far beyond the specific settings in which the research teams are working.

Many of the conditions individuals experience when they are young children continue to influence their health and well-being much later in their lives. For example, research evidence has demonstrated that children enrolled in high-quality preschools are more likely to attend college and have full-time employment as adults (Reynolds et al. 2007). Children who are obese before age five are more likely to be obese later in adolescence (Nader et al. 2006) and into adulthood (Simmons et al. 2016). Adverse Childhood Experiences (ACEs) experienced before age five are associated with negative mental health outcomes into adulthood (Herzog and Schmahl 2018). With the long-term goal of building a culture of health, the Robert Wood Johnson Foundation's Interdisciplinary Research Leaders (IRL) program made early childhood health a target area for their first cohort of the program. In bringing together community members working to promote the health and well-being of young children and researchers well-versed in evaluation and knowledge creation, the IRL program sought to fuel research that would not only add foundational evidence for early childhood intervention efforts but also grow a cohort of leaders prepared to cut across professional silos and take on the inherent challenges of early childhood health head on. Although community-academic partnerships around early childhood are not unheard of (e.g., Tribal Early Childhood Research Center; Whitesell et al. 2015; CBPR in Early HeadStart; McAllister et al. 2003), collaborations that bridge the gap between "ivory tower" early childhood education research and community institutions serving young children are not the norm. By working together on collaborative, community-informed research, the IRL teams aim to shift policies and systems that will affect child health. For example, authors describe projects focused on the birth experiences of women at high risk for negative birth outcomes, interventions focused on parenting infants and preschool education, and research that will change systems of Women, Infants, and Children (WIC) education delivery and child welfare/healthcare communication.

The Structure of the Volume

The chapters in this volume discuss how community-engaged research on very profound and challenging topics within early childhood health is currently being conducted throughout the United States. The scope of academics and community partners engaging in this work is incredibly diverse. Academic partners authoring chapters in this volume represent public health, psychology, policy, economics, medicine, nutrition, and geography researchers. Community partners include not only grassroots partners, such as community organizers and community residents, but also representatives from communities of policy and practice, such as medical practioners, nonprofit leaders, and policymakers. The chapters illustrate how teams of community partners and researchers can, and have, bonded to overcome the challenges of doing community-engaged research well, because they care deeply about the promoting the health of young children in their communities and they feel that evidence-based research for change is key. The authors share why they are pursuing this research and how joining the effort to build a culture of health through interdisciplinary and community-engaged research has impacted them and their work.

Despite covering diverse geographic areas, research projects, and experiences, the chapters in this volume are structured in a similar way. They outline what the research team wanted to work on as they set out to conduct community-engaged research, how they went about doing it, the stumbling blocks and supports they found as they engaged in the research process, and the results of their efforts. The first team research chapter, "Enhancing the Arkansas Birthing Project through Technology," orients our empirical focus to very early childhood interventions to promote health and the development of the Arkansas Birthing Project. The research team supported a volunteer peer-mentoring program for women of color during pregnancy and the first year of each baby's life. Ensuring social and community support for these women, as well as standardized education with the use of technology, were parts of the team's joint effort. Chapter 3, "A Place-Based Approach to Early Childhood Wellness in Cincinnati: Communities Acting for Kids Empowerment (CAKE)," centers neighborhood organizing in Cincinnati, Ohio, following a resident-driven tax aimed at providing universal preschool. The team—consisting of a health geographer, a clinical psychologist, and a community organizer—used community organizing in the Carthage and Roselawn neighborhoods to build resident leadership and power. Using participatory research methods, the team organized community meetings to identify community priorities for early childhood wellness. Chapter 4, "Finding Our Way as a Cross-Systems Team: Lessons Learned from an Interdisciplinary Research Team," outlines the work of an Indiana–based research team, consisting of a psychology professor, an education researcher, and a community organizer. Together they worked to promote social and emotional health and developmental well-being in early childhood. Specifically, they were interested in addressing the health impacts of mass incarceration on children in the state. The team reflected on their experience of bringing together both academics and community-based institutions around the issue of access to high-quality pre-k education for children whose caregivers experienced incarceration. Recognizing the importance of structural racism in unequal health outcomes, chapter 5, "Improving Racial Equity in Birth Outcomes: A Community-Based, Culturally Centered Approach," features the work by two public health professors and the owner of a for-profit birthing center in Minneapolis. The authors described the core content, experiences, and outcomes of pregnancy and childbirth care provided to clients by a culturally competent, African American–owned birth center: Roots Community Birth Center. The team outlined how their work reveals a new model of care that allows for the healing of both personal and historical trauma. Chapter 6, "Creating Transformational Nonprofit/University Partnerships in Public Health: Lessons Derived from Collaboration between Room to Grow and Columbia University," features the Columbia Study of Mothers and Babies, an exploratory randomized controlled trial of the Room to Grow program model. Room to Grow is a therapeutic, strengths-based program, where the provision of items is designed to improve personalized parenting goals aligned with the program's three-year curriculum. Chapter 7, "Building Strong Partnerships with the Puerto Rico WIC Program for Promoting Healthy Lifestyles in Early Childhood and a Long-Lasting Culture of Health," discusses the planned transformation of the Puerto Rico WIC program, aimed at promoting healthy lifestyles in early childhood and a long-lasting culture of health for Puerto Rican families. The study of this federal program's adaptation in Puerto Rico took a sharp turn in September 2017 when the island suffered catastrophic damage and loss of life after Hurricanes Irma and Maria. The team shifted their work to assess how WIC service continuity and needs assessments were secured in the wake of a major disaster on an island where most of the food is imported.

The final empirical chapter, "In Search of Child Welfare and Child Health Collaboration," presents the team research of a child abuse pediatrician, a public policy professor, and the deputy director of Utah's child welfare agency. The team looked into policies and practices that support collaboration between child welfare and child health professionals in cases where infants may be abused and neglected. Taking lessons from professionals working in highly collaborative states, the team assessed the implementation of collaborative policies and practices in Utah with an aim to improve interprofessional collaboration and health outcomes for infants. Chapter 9, "Interdisciplinary Community-Engaged Research (ICER) for Health: Growing in Understanding and Effectiveness," brings together the experiences and insights shared by authors, drawing out commonalities and distinct lessons learned with regard to these teams' community-engaged research for better health. Chapter 9 also examines the crosscutting benefits and challenges of community-engaged research on issues related to early childhood health as exemplified by these teams' efforts.

Paving the Way:
Road Maps for Interdisciplinary Community-Engaged Research

This book should be of interest to scholars and practitioners working across diverse disciplines and in a multitude of community settings. Anyone interested in going into public health, community health, and early childhood health—particularly for at-risk children—will find this volume to be very valuable. It provides examples of cutting-edge research being done in these areas of interest and practice. Practitioners who are considering doing an assessment of a current program, designing a new service or intervention, or figuring out what works, can turn to this volume as a road map for building collaboration with researchers.

Researchers need community engagement to do research; disseminate knowledge about research findings; and implement evidence-based interventions, programs, and policies. We know from decades of experience that the traditional top-down approach to studying groups, populations, and communities does very little to change actual practices in real-world settings. In order to understand how to work together most effectively, however, scholars, practitioners, and community organizations could use a road map. Researchers and community partners need to collaborate to understand how to ask scientifically rigorous questions that are informed by community experiences and how to develop evidence-based interventions and programs that fit the community context. The community needs to be involved from the beginning in order to build community buy-in into the research that is conducted "on them" if we are going to effectively address social determinants of health and find local solutions to global challenges. Our hope is that scholars who are interested in effective community engagement and partnering in research will find in this volume examples of good practice that will get them going on this imperative but challenging work.

Students learning research methods aimed at answering pressing questions about social problems should also read this volume. For these students this volume serves as an applied methods text, exemplifying and hopefully generating fruitful discussions about the strengths and weaknesses of participatory methods and the messiness of community engagement in what is often assumed to be an objective and clinical research process. It can also serve as a good text on action research and an example of applied quantitative methods. For doctoral students getting ready to do fieldwork or design their own community-engaged research dissertation, this volume should serve as an excellent specialized methods primer and field preparation guide. Finally, for individual researchers or research teams looking to apply for grants for team-based research and/ or community-based research, this volume presents excellent examples and research guidance.

Most of all, as editors of this book, we hope this volume will inspire you as an engaged community member, as a researcher, organizer, or possible community partner to pursue community-engaged research and continue to move important work on health, equity, justice, and community forward.

References

Balazs, C. L., and R. Morello-Frosch. 2013. "The Three Rs: How Community-Based Participatory Research Strengthens the Rigor, Relevance, and Reach of Science." *Environmental Justice* 6 (1): 9–16.

Clinical and Translational Science Awards Consortium (CTSA) and Community Engagement Key Function Committee Task Force on the Principles of Community Engagement. 2011. *Principles of Community Engagement.* 2nd ed. NIH Publication no. 11-778. Bethesda, MD: National Institutes of Health. https://www.atsdr.cdc.gov/communityengagement/pdf/PCE_Report_508 _FINAL.pdf.

Cyril, S., B. J. Smith, A. Possamai-Inesedy, and A. M. Renzaho. 2015. "Exploring the Role of Community Engagement in Improving the Health of Disadvantaged Populations: A Systematic Review." *Global Health Action* 8 (1): 1–12. doi: 10.3402/gha.v8.29842.

Drahota, A., R. D. Meza, B. Brikho, M. Naaf, J. A. Estabillo, E. D. Gomez, S. F. Vejnoska, S. Dufek, A. C. Stahmer, and G. A. Aarons. 2016. "Community-Academic Partnerships: A Systematic Review of the State of the Literature and Recommendations for Future Research." *Milbank Quarterly* 94 (1): 163–214.

Driscoll, A. 2008. "Carnegie's Community-Engagement Classification: Intentions and Insights." *Change: The Magazine of Higher Learning* 40 (1): 38–41.

George, A. S., V. Mehra, K. Scott, and V. Sriram. 2015. "Community Participation in Health Systems Research: A Systematic Review Assessing the State of Research, the Nature of Interventions Involved and the Features of Engagement with Communities." *PLoS ONE* 10 (10): 1–25. doi: 10.1371/journal.pone.0141091.

Herzog, J. I., and C. Schmahl. 2018. "Adverse Childhood Experiences and the Consequences on Neurobiological, Psychosocial, and Somatic Conditions across the Lifespan." *Frontiers in Psychiatry* 9:420. doi: 10.3389/fpsyt.2018.00420.

Nader, P. R., M. O'Brien, R. Houts, R. Bradley, J. Belsky, R. Crosnoe, and E. J. Susman. 2006. "Identifying Risk for Obesity in Early Childhood." *Pediatrics* 118 (3): e594–e601.

Oetzel, J. G., N. Wallerstein, B. Duran, S. Sanchez-Youngman, T. Nguyen, K. Woo, and M. Alegria. 2018. "Impact of Participatory Health Research: A Test of the Community-Based Participatory Research Conceptual Model." *BioMed Research International*, 1–12. doi: 10.1155/2018/7281405.

O'Mara-Eves, A., G. Brunton, G. McDaid, S. Oliver, J. Kavanagh, F. Jamal, and J. Thomas. 2013. "Community Engagement to Reduce Inequalities in Health: A Systematic Review, Meta-Analysis and Economic Analysis." *Public Health Research* 1 (4).

Patient-Centered Outcomes Research Center (PCORI). https://www.pcori.org/.

Reynolds, A. J., J. A. Temple, S. R. Ou, D. L. Robertson, J. P. Mersky, J. W. Topitzes, and M. D. Niles. 2007. "Effects of a School-Based, Early Childhood Intervention on Adult Health and Well-Being: A 19-Year Follow-Up of Low-Income Families." *Archives of Pediatrics and Adolescent Medicine* 161 (8): 730–39.

Rifkin, S. B. 2014. "Examining the Links between Community Participation and Health Outcomes: A Review of the Literature." *Health Policy and Planning* 29 (2): ii98–ii106. doi: 10.1093/heapol/czu076.

Sarrami-Foroushani, P., J. Travaglia, D. Debono, and J. Braithwaite. 2014. "Key Concepts in Consumer and Community Engagement: A Scoping Meta-Review." *BMC Health Services Research* 14 (1): 1–9.

Simmonds, M., A. Llewellyn, C. G. Owen, and N. Woolacott. 2016. "Predicting Adult Obesity from Childhood Obesity: A Systematic Review and Meta-Analysis." *Obesity Reviews* 17 (2): 95–107.

South, J., A. M. Bagnall, J. A. Stansfield, K. J. Southby, and P. Mehta. 2017. "An Evidence-Based Framework on Community-Centred Approaches for Health: England, UK." *Health Promotion International* 34 (2): 356–66. doi: 10.1093/heapro/dax083.

Winer, M., and K. Ray. 1994. *Collaboration Handbook: Creating, Sustaining, and Enjoying the Journey*. St. Paul, MN: Amherst H. Wilder Foundation.

World Health Organization (WHO) Regional Office for Europe. 2012. *Health 2020: A European Policy Framework Supporting Action across Government and Society for Health and Well-Being*. Copenhagen: WHO Regional Office for Europe. http://www.euro.who.int/__data/assets/pdf_file/0011/199532/Health2020-Long.pdf.

World Health Organization (WHO). 2016. "Shanghai Declaration on Promoting Health in the 2030 Agenda for Sustainable Development." Delivered at the Ninth Global Conference on Health Promotion, November 21, Shanghai, China.

Chapter 2

Enhancing the Arkansas Birthing Project through Technology

Sarah Rhoads
University of Tennessee Health Science Center

Zenobia Harris
Arkansas Birthing Project

Hari Eswaran
University of Arkansas for Medical Sciences

Chapter Context

Zenobia Harris: I have always embraced being a change agent in public health. This experience gave me an opportunity to engage in research that could have an impact on a nationwide network of change enablers for improved perinatal outcomes for women of color.

Sarah Rhodes: Since I began as a nurse on labor and delivery, I have had a passion for improving maternal and neonatal outcomes. There is not one simple solution for improving outcomes. Partnering with the community and the Arkansas Birthing Project has been a wonderful experience to learn more about the nonmedical needs of women and their families during pregnancy and after birth.

Hari Eswaran: I have worked in the area of prenatal monitoring and obstetrics for the past twenty years. With my background in technology and research, my desire has always been to find ways to utilize technology to work toward improving maternal child health. Collaborating with the community partner really helped me understand the community perspective, which enabled me to tailor the technology to the needs.

The Arkansas Birthing Project is well established in Arkansas and part of a larger organization—Birthing Project USA—which has been supporting women and families for over thirty years. Our research collaboration enables us to combine these established programs with the tele-health and educational infrastructure the academic medical center has developed.

Introduction

The Mississippi Delta region of the United States is comprised of the southern sections of Mississippi, Arkansas, and Louisiana. Because of its unique racial, cultural, and economic history, this part of the United States has been characterized as the most southern part of the American South. It was developed as one of the richest cotton-growing areas in the nation before the Civil War. The land was developed along the river-fronts for cotton plantations, which were dependent on the labor of black slaves, who comprised the vast majority of the population in this area before the Civil War. Widespread poverty and numerous health ailments affect the progeny—black and white—of many of the original inhabitants of this region of the United States.

Many researchers have come to the Mississippi Delta region to "help" the communities—families, men, women, and children—who live in this area of the United States. Healthcare providers and researchers often want to implement programs and special projects to improve maternal and neonatal outcomes. Researchers have a variety of ideas and methods by which they believe health outcomes can be improved. This is particularly true when research involves examining and deciphering long-standing, recalcitrant health and mortality issues affecting maternal and child health populations in the Delta. Many of these researchers have a commitment to the area; others are seeking the next grant or funding opportunity and the potential for celebrity status associated with them. Often the most idealistic of intentions will result in a short, brief intervention done "to" or "for" the women or the community. The results are disseminated in a research journal and the intervention goes away at the completion of the grant funding, regardless of positive or negative findings. Many of the community members are wary of being the subjects of research projects. They are tired of being told what is best for them from researchers outside the community, and by researchers who cannot relate to their day-to-day life. How is our project different? Our project—the Arkansas Birthing Project, an affiliate of Birthing Project USA—is a community-based and community-led mentoring program that provides social and emotional support to women during pregnancy and for one year after the birth of their baby. The beauty of the program is that it begins in, resides in, and is led by the community where the woman resides. It is proving to be a successful way to encourage and support grassroots empowerment of people who have been victims of poor intergenerational health and wealth status.

Research Team Collaboration

How does a research team come together? That can be a complex and complicated question. This is the first time all the individuals of our team have worked together. Each team member has a different focus, but we collectively collaborate to address health concerns. Zenobia Harris has a background in maternal and child health nursing, a wealth of community health supporters and public health knowledge, and serves as our team's community partner. Sarah Rhoads has a connected health technology background as well as extensive maternal/child nursing experience. Hari Eswaran is a basic science researcher who uses new and novel technology to examine health outcomes. The Robert Wood Johnson Foundation program—Interdisciplinary Research Leaders (IRL)—is what brought us all together as a team. The IRL program has challenged us as fellows to examine our own personal experiences and biases as well as the community, social, and structural biases that affect us where we live and work. This allows us to openly examine the issues and dialogue related to gender and racial bias, health inequities, southern culture, slavery, availability and access to healthcare and social supports, and many other related issues. It has also taught us to trust our partnership with each other. This took us each a while to learn, but has been worth our many team-building meetings, discussions, and outreach efforts, and ultimately involved reaching out to each other as friends with many different life experiences. Each of us has taken different paths to get to where we are today.

Zenobia Harris is African American, was born in Arkansas, was raised in California, and returned to Arkansas to attend college, work as a public health nurse practitioner, and ultimately become a public health administrator. She is currently serving as executive director of the Arkansas Birthing Project after having served in various roles in the public health system of Arkansas for over thirty years. Hari Eswaran is originally from India, traveled to the United States to attend graduate school in Mississippi, and moved to Arkansas to earn a doctorate. He has remained in Arkansas for the past twenty-five years and is currently a researcher in the Department of Obstetrics and Gynecology at the University of Arkansas for Medical Sciences. Sarah Rhoads is white, was born in Arkansas, is a first-generation college student, and has a twenty-plus-year nursing history with a focus in maternal child health. She currently serves as a professor of nursing in the Department of Health Promotion and Disease Prevention at the University of Tennessee Health Science Center. Even though the personal and professional experiences that led to our collaboration are different, we come together to examine women's, maternal, and child health needs and experiences in Arkansas. The three of us are very focused on strategies that can add maximum benefit to women's and children's health, using interventions that are not costly financially and are culturally congruent within the unique spaces occupied by Arkansas women.

Community Partner

Zenobia Harris is the executive director of the Arkansas Birthing Project. The Arkansas Birthing Project is an affiliate of Birthing Project USA (BPUSA). Birthing Project USA: The Underground Railroad to New Life is a volunteer peer-based mentoring program that has served women and their babies for over thirty years related to healthcare and social support. The BPUSA's main mission is to encourage better outcomes for mothers and babies by providing practical support for women during pregnancy and for one year after the birth of the baby. The program was founded in 1988 by Kathryn Hall-Trujillo—an Arkansas native—while she was working as a fiscal administrator for the California State Department of Health. It is one of a few original maternal and child health programs in the country that was created by an African American woman to support African American women and their babies. The program is often called the "underground railroad" of our times, aiding women on their pregnancy and parenting journeys. The program helps women become "free" to the point of functioning in today's society, and during that process leads other women to "freedom" one step at a time. Because of the local and community nature of the program, it helps women link to local services and programs.

The Birthing Project USA recruits local community women and supports them to serve as peer mentors called Sister Friends. These women are the guides for pregnant women on the journey to "freedom." The pregnant women receiving peer support are endearingly called Little Sisters. The women are grouped together in groups of ten by a local project or Bunch manager according to personal preferences and the Little Sister's delivery date. Each group of ten Little Sisters and ten Sister Friends is called a Bunch. The Sister Friends mentor the Little Sisters during pregnancy and for the first year of the baby's life—usually about a fifteen- to eighteen-month period all together. The Big Sister–Little Sister pair is required to connect with each other for about eight to ten hours a month. Oftentimes they use text messaging or in-person visits for these mentoring connections. The Sister Friends are guided by a Bunch manager, who meets with the Sister Friends on a monthly basis providing educational information and support. During monthly Sister Friend meetings, the Bunch manager checks in on the Sister Friends and sees how they are doing as well as receives updates on the Little Sister's status. The Sister Friends are required to be three very important things: responsible, compassionate, and committed. The Birthing Project USA training manual describes the volunteer mentor job functions as: ensuring the Little Sister has a prenatal provider and is going to her appointments, assisting the Little Sister in understanding instructions received from her healthcare provider, making sure the Little Sister has a way to get to medical appointments and has access to childcare if needed, and identifying and connecting the Little Sister with any needed support services. The Sister Friend attends the monthly meetings and receives needed support and guidance from the Bunch manager. The Bunch manager advises all Sister Friends to avoid giving medical advice, transporting the Little Sister (especially if they do not have auto insurance), or making the Little Sister dependent on them. Ideally the Sister Friend attends at least one prenatal visit with the Little Sister and plans to be present at the hospital with her Little Sister during the birth of her baby. Sister Friends are not required to be in the birthing room during the delivery, but they can provide important support before, during, and/or after birth in many ways.

One of the most endearing and noteworthy aspects of Birthing Project USA is how it is grounded in the cultural heritage and traditions of the African American community. Many of the trainings and meetings begin with testifying—an old tradition in the black church whereby members express their gratitude for their lives and those of their loved ones. This tradition serves as a source of hope and strength for the community and doubles as a unifying call within the extended family structure of the Birthing Project USA. The Sister Friends and Little Sisters come together to celebrate milestones of the pregnancy and the baby's life during the course of their mentoring relationship. Several celebratory events occur, such as baby showers and birthday parties for the babies. At one event in particular, the dreaming ceremony, the Sister Friends and Little Sisters come together as a group and talk about the future they dream of for the baby. They create a human circle and allow each member of the circle to take turns describing their dreams and positive affirmations in a whispered tone to the mother and her baby as they circle the human circle in the room.

Birthing Project USA's mission is "to improve women's health and birth outcomes through SisterFriending ™, education, community collaboration, and capacity building" (https://www.birthingprojectusa.org/index.html). Operating in many US cities and several foreign counties, including Malawi and Cuba, at any one time, BPUSA has improved the chances for black babies to be born healthy. The founder of this growing global organization, Kathryn Hall-Trujillo, is an Ashoka global social entrepreneur. Social entrepreneurs are individuals with innovative solutions to society's most pressing social, cultural, and environmental challenges. They are ambitious and persistent in examining major issues and offering new ideas for systems-level change. The Ashoka organization identifies and supports the world's leading social entrepreneurs. In the words of Hall-Trujillo, BPUSA "is in the business of birth. We know it is a natural occurrence. We also know that it takes focus and assistance, is comprised of stages and transitions and is full of mystery and magic.... We respect the value and contribution of each individual to be a part of defining problems and solutions, participate in building and visualizing a better world, and to be involved in creating an organization that works for them" (Hall-Trujillo 2019). It is our hope to enhance the birth experiences of black women in Arkansas through enhancing the Birthing Project model using modern-day technology to improve the education, training, and mentoring experiences of program participants.

Research Idea

Sarah Rhoads has worked with both Zenobia Harris and Hari Eswaran on several projects over the years; she was the magnet that pulled our team together. She proposed that we work on a research project where each member could utilize their varied experiences and address interests that could have a meaningful impact on the development of a culture of health in Arkansas and, potentially, nationally through BPUSA. The Birthing Project is well established in Arkansas, so it was a challenge to come up with a research idea that would continue the legacy of the program and not interfere with the community-led piece of the intervention. Ultimately our team decided to explore the use of technology to expand the program's reach. Rhoads and the education team at the Center for Distance Health at the University of Arkansas for Medical Sciences had already created interactive educational modules and a website portal for childbirth education, safe sleep, car seat safety, birth control options, breastfeeding, as well as many other topics (patientslearn.org). Our research team mused over whether we could use these interactive modules within the Bunches to enhance the education and knowledge of Sister Friends and Little Sisters. With a volunteer-based program like the Birthing Project, many volunteers do not have a background in maternal/child health but will rely on their own personal experiences. Since the Birthing Project is a social support program, it provides and examines the social aspects related to a healthy pregnancy, birth, and child-rearing, such as access to food, transportation, housing, and other essential needs. It does not focus on providing medical interventions, advice, or education. Even though the focus of the program is social support, the need for accurate health information relayed from the Sister Friends to the Little Sisters is still a very important factor contributing to improved health outcomes. Historically there has been a training process for Sister Friends regarding health information during pregnancy, childbirth, and care of the baby during the first year of life, but it has not been quantified from Birthing Project to Birthing Project. Our research question is: "Can we utilize technology to educate Sister Friends and Little Sisters about health information without losing the personal nature of this program?"

Research Methods

We divided up the research project into two different phases. During the first phase, we interviewed former Sister Friends and Little Sisters using focus groups to gather their perceptions about their experiences in the program. We asked about the challenging and rewarding parts of the program. We also asked them about the use of technology to provide the education and assess if they would use the information in the educational modules and on the web portal if given the opportunity to do so. The second phase is being conducted with four Bunches—two randomly selected rural and two randomly selected urban Bunches. Each Bunch is assigned to either a "technology" group or a "non-technology" group. Upon enrollment in the program and at the first meeting, the Sister Friends and Little Sisters complete demographic and baseline surveys. After completing the surveys—dependent on which group they are members of—they are either given tablets with the educational modules or a book about pregnancy and baby care. Post-treatment surveys will be conducted eight weeks after the last Little Sister in each Bunch has delivered her baby. At that time, a focus group will be facilitated to gather the collective thoughts of all the Sister Friends and Little Sisters about the use of the technology in disseminating information.

Research Challenges and Successes

As with any research team and project, we have experienced several challenges. One of the greatest challenges our team has experienced is time availability. All three of us have various professional and personal responsibilities that take us in many different directions on a daily basis. In the short time we have been working together as a team, we have encountered many personal roadblocks as well as professional hurdles. Juggling personal and professional lives while participating in a time-intensive fellowship and conducting a research study has proven difficult at times. To assist with the project, we have reached out to include other team members, such as a research assistant to assist with data collection and an academic researcher to assist with data analysis.

The use of technology has also been shown to be problematic during our project. Initially we were advised by the instructional designers that the online educational modules could be downloaded and accessed without using Wi-Fi or cellular data. After the tablets were purchased and the modules were downloaded, this proved to be false. This has created access issues related to the educational modules, especially for Sister Friends in the rural settings, where access to free Wi-Fi is scarce. Another barrier we have encountered has been deciding between using android tablets and iPads for the participants. We had to hire an information technology support person to assist with creating folders on the tablets' home screens to ensure they were easily accessed once the Sister Friend had access to Wi-Fi. An additional workaround for this issue was asking the Sister Friends and Little Sisters to download the mobile-friendly website to their home screen to enable them to log onto the website and access the educational content with a few clicks. Even if the Sister Friends and Little Sisters have the website saved on the home screen of their device, they would need cellular data or a Wi-Fi signal to retrieve the modules. Many of the Sister Friends and Little Sisters do not have unlimited data plans and therefore cannot readily access the modules.

Many of the Sister Friends have numerous professional and personal responsibilities. They struggle to make the monthly meetings due to their busy lives, and oftentimes at the meetings that are attended the Sister Friends appear very tired; some even appear overwhelmed with life's responsibilities. The Bunch meetings are a safe place where Sister Friends can communicate with the Bunch manager and each other, and discuss not only issues their Little Sister is having but also issues in their own day-to-day lives. This support system for the Sister Friend is a benefit to her as well as to the Little Sister.

A great bond has been developed between our team members. We often benefit from discussions about research, women's health, African American heritage, southern heritage, and the United States' history of slavery and racial segregation. Our team engages in difficult discussions about why African American women currently have high rates of maternal and infant mortality and morbidity. We have agreed to embrace the Institute for Perinatal Quality Improvement's initiative—known as SPEAK UP for African American and Black Women and SPEAK UP Against Racism—in an attempt to make other healthcare professionals aware of the maternal mortality and morbidity disparities experienced by women of color (www.perinatalqi.org). There is a profound need to promote greater awareness of this incidence and to urge actions to decrease this incidence. These discussions have allowed us to grow both personally and professionally. Our team now looks at the healthcare system and research studies with a different perspective after these in-depth discussions.

Dissemination of Research Collaboration

Rhoads, Harris, and Eswaran have submitted multiple abstracts for presentation at regional and national conferences. The primary purpose of dissemination is to present information about the Arkansas Birthing Project and Birthing Project USA to a variety of healthcare and community audiences—public health nurses, maternal/infant nurses, public health administrators, and public health practitioners. Reflecting after the last presentation we offered at the Association of Women's Health, Obstetrical and Neonatal Nurses, we realized Harris has a special gift for listening and responding to others. After our presentations, people from the audience flocked to her to tell their birth stories or the birth story of a person close to them. Some women discuss their lack of support during their own pregnancy; some talk about how they are mentoring young women who are currently pregnant; others want to start a Birthing Project in their community, church, or town. Harris listens, supports, and validates each woman's experience. One woman—a nurse herself—discussed how she was supporting her niece, who had recently become pregnant and who lived in a challenging, unsupportive environment. She then proceeded to give an in-depth description of her personal experience as a teen mother and the struggles she had when she was pregnant and delivered her baby. Today she lives in a rural community in the South and works as a labor and delivery nurse. She wants to start a Birthing Project in her church to give back—to help and support other young women in her community who may be experiencing a rough time, as she did. This and many similar stories were shared with Harris over and over again. Harris realizes that personal pregnancy experiences and challenges can inspire some women to give support to other women, especially those who are pregnant. It is our dream to share our research data with the larger BPUSA organization in hopes of routinely incorporating the use of technology-assisted educational messages into the standard training offered to Sister Friends across the many Birthing Projects established in the United States and abroad. Magnifying the voices of the women telling their story and serving their desire to give back to their local community builds on the overall premise of the Birthing Project USA—"I am my sister's keeper." We are proud to be a part of this storytelling, empowering experience, which helps to give another voice to the voiceless.

References

Hall-Trujillo, K. 2019. "A Word from the Founder." Birthing Project USA, http://www.birthingprojectusa.org/a-word-from-the-founder.html.

Chapter 3

A Place-Based Approach
to Early Childhood Wellness in Cincinnati

Communities Acting for Kids Empowerment (CAKE)

Michael Topmiller
American Academy of Family Physicians

Farrah Jacquez
University of Cincinatti

Jamie-Lee Morris
Elementz

Chapter Context

Farrah Jacquez: As a traditionally trained clinical psychologist, I spent a lot of time doing research on children and families to understand mental illness. Discovering community-based participatory research changed my entire value system and focused my efforts on working with—instead of on—children and families to make real-world change.

Michael Topmiller: My reasons for pursuing this work stem directly from my experiences in failed community-based participatory research projects where I learned the value of community buy-in and trust, the need for research questions and priorities to come directly from the community, and finally, the need for tangible results that the community can own and use to advocate for change.

Jamie-Lee Morris: My experience in community organizing exposed me to many different approaches to create local change. The opportunity to explore nontraditional approaches to collaborating with community in a way that gives them agency to take on leadership roles in the process has been the most rewarding.

Together our objective is to ensure that every child has the opportunity to have the happy and healthy life they deserve. To do this, we want to ensure every child has access to resources in their community, such as high-quality early childhood education. Ensuring the well-being of children in our neighborhoods required engaging parents, early childhood education providers, and other local stakeholders as co-researchers, and having them co-lead and guide the research. Our team sought to build a network of early childhood health advocates that would be able to gather insights from our neighborhoods on multiple levels, identify local assets and resources, and take action that directly reflects community priorities and enhances existing assets. To build our network and reach our goals, we needed to involve our community partners as co-researchers, which meant giving them equal voice and power within the collaboration, involving them in every step of the research process, and having them lead our action and dissemination aspects of the project.

The resulting partnership, Communities Acting for Kids Empowerment (CAKE), ended up as a hybrid community advisory board (CAB)–co-researcher model where community partners played a variety of roles as part of our team. All CAKE partners were involved with making decisions and guiding research priorities, but some members played more active roles in data collection, analysis, and interpretation. We learned significant lessons from our experience working within this hybrid model for doing community-based participatory research. In the formation stage of our collaboration, we learned the importance of formalizing roles and responsibilities and balancing the representation of diverse community voices with the formation of a clear and distinct narrative. In the operations stage of collaborating, we learned the importance of establishing decision-making and communication processes. In the maintenance stage, we identified the importance of group self-evaluation and in appreciating new and developing roles as partnerships grow and change.

Communities Acting for Kids Empowerment (CAKE) is a community-academic partnership focused on early childhood wellness in Carthage and Roselawn, two neighborhoods in northern Cincinnati. CAKE is led by three Robert Wood Johnson Foundation Interdisciplinary Research Leader (IRL) fellows, including a community organizer from a local Baptist church, a research geographer focused on health equity, and a psychology professor at a research university. Together the three developed CAKE as the infrastructure to guide research that represents the community voice and has a high potential for impact. In this chapter, we describe CAKE as a model for community-academic partnerships that integrates two existing models in the literature: community advisory boards (CABs) and the community member co-researcher. In our CAB–co-researcher hybrid model of doing community-engaged research, local early childhood stakeholders were recruited to be part of a leadership team to highlight assets, identify needs, and develop a multilevel intervention to improve early childhood wellness in Carthage and Roselawn. We discuss how the CAB–co-researcher hybrid model has functioned during the formation, operation, and maintenance of our project.

The community advisory board (CAB) model has been widely used in community-engaged research. CABs are formalized structures for community-academic partnerships that provide the infrastructure for allowing community input, advice, and priorities into research projects (Israel et al. 1998). Community-based participatory research projects (CBPR) using the CAB are diverse; examples include a six-member CAB focused on improving mobility and access for people with spinal cord injuries (Newman et al. 2009), and an eight-member CAB made up of housing officials, community members, and members of local organizations focused on smoking cessation in public housing (Andrews et al. 2007). The extent to which community members influence the direction of research depends on their level of engagement with the CAB. In some CABs, the role of community participants is as advisors, where the power and ultimately decision-making are left to research partners (Morin et al. 2003). In co-researcher models—also called peer researcher, lay researcher, and insider researcher models—community members are equal partners in the research, with assigned leadership positions and decision-making powers (Vaughn et al. 2018). Practitioners of the co-researcher model describe how community members are involved in every step of the research process, including the development of heuristic models that guide entire projects (Allen et al. 2006) and carrying out data collection and analysis (Jacquez et al. 2018). The co-researcher model has the potential to significantly improve both the quality and the relevance of research by producing hybrid knowledge (Brookes 2006) that equally values both the lived experience expertise of community researchers and the scientific expertise of academic researchers as required elements in the research process. A review of ten years of co-researcher model literature identified improved prevention, improved health and social services, community capacity-building/empowerment, and improved research methodology development as their most-cited benefits (Vaughn et al. 2018).

Newman and colleagues provide guidance on the best processes of CABs, focusing on three domains: formation, operation, and maintenance (Newman et al. 2011). Formation occurs at the beginning stages of a CAB, where the purpose, roles, and functions of the CAB are clearly defined. A key aspect of the formation stage is defining the role of the CAB as advisors (providing guidance, but not part of decision-making) or partners (shared power, decision-making). A second major component of the formation phase is the composition of its members, including decisions around identifying and recruiting members based on specific criteria. The operation domain of CABs involves establishing operating principles for how the community-academic partnership is going to work. These include defining leadership roles, power structure, and decision-making criteria and protocol. While the formation phase may define the role of CABs as partners, the operation phase explicitly describes the process of how it is going to work. The final major process component of CABs is maintenance, which includes evaluating the work of CABs and plans for sustainability.

Using Newman et al.'s (2011) best processes for CABs as a guide, this chapter describes the key processes involved with our CAB–co-researcher hybrid model, focusing on successful elements, innovations, and areas needing improvement. We begin by providing an overview of the origin, goals, and geographic focus of Communities Acting for Kids Empowerment (CAKE). Next we describe the key processes, including the selection and recruitment of CAKE members, meeting schedules, decision-making structure, self-evaluation, and plans for sustainability, in the context of the three domains of successful CABs. We conclude with lessons learned and reflections for future community-academic partnerships.

Overview of Communities Acting for Kids Empowerment (CAKE)

CAKE's origins stem from the Robert Wood Johnson Interdisciplinary Research Leaders (IRL) program, a three-year fellowship program that teams two researchers with a community partner to conduct community-engaged research. The three IRL fellows (this chapter's authors), henceforth referred to as IR leaders, were awarded the fellowship and research funding based on a proposal to use a place-based, asset-focused approach to improve early childhood wellness. One of the key elements of the proposal was to establish a community leadership team using a CAB–co-researcher hybrid model, where community stakeholders were active partners with the IR leaders and had shared decision-making power. The leadership team was charged with achieving three key aims: (1) creating a network of engaged community members, education providers, and stakeholders ready for action; (2) raising awareness in Carthage and Roselawn of preschool opportunities and benefits; and (3) developing a multi-level intervention with systematic input from across community sectors.

CAKE's focus on early childhood wellness was sparked by grassroots effort to expand access to quality preschool in Cincinnati. Cincinnati Preschool Promise, the 501c3 organization charged with implementing universal preschool, passed in a landslide in November 2016 as a merged campaign with grassroots leaders and the local Cincinnati Public School District (Cincinnati Preschool Promise, CPP). This was a historical win for the community given the collaboration between the local school levy and a grassroots effort joining forces for children. The timing of preschool expansion created a unique opportunity to engage community leaders and neighborhood residents into evidence-based action to promote early childhood wellness and provided an opportunity for us to hold accountable those responsible for distributing the funds, ensuring that it reaches the families most in need.

There are three major reasons why CAKE focused its efforts on Carthage and Roselawn. First, the IR leaders wanted to focus efforts on specific neighborhoods as part of a place-based approach. Place-based approaches address health disparities by engaging community stakeholders in a specified geography to improve community conditions and promote optimal health outcomes (Dankwa-Mullen and Perez-Stable 2016). Unlike traditional research that focuses on one system, place-based

approaches address the multiple contexts that contribute to negative outcomes in early childhood—individual, family, school, and community.
Second, Carthage and Roselawn are representative of vulnerable communities across Cincinnati, yet they are geographically separate and lack
access to medical and higher education resources in the city. In a city
that has one of the highest childhood poverty rates in the United States
(US Census Bureau 2012–2016), children in Carthage and Roselawn are
especially vulnerable. Half of the children in these neighborhoods live
in poverty, and 99 percent of children in neighborhood public schools
are eligible for free or reduced lunch (National Center for Education
Statistics 2015–2016). While the majority of Roselawn's seven thousand
residents are African American (82 percent), Carthage has a diverse
population—about one-fifth of its almost three thousand residents are
African American and more than one-fourth are Latino, one of the
highest concentrations of Latinos in the Cincinnati area (US Census
Bureau 2012–2016). The final reason is that two of the IR leaders already
had strong connections to the two neighborhoods. Farrah Jacquez has
been working in Roselawn for seven years with the school with the
largest population of Latino children in Cincinnati and with Su Casa
Hispanic Center, the social service agency that is the primary provider
of social services for Latino immigrants in Cincinnati. While working as
a community organizer, Jamie-Lee Morris regularly collaborated with
two local churches in the area, Carthage Christian Church and New
Prospect Baptist Church, that have already organized around universal
preschool and are actively working on community development projects
in the two neighborhoods.

The initial proposal of the IR leaders included a variety of research
activities focused on identifying assets and barriers related to early
childhood wellness in the two neighborhoods, including participatory

focus groups (which we refer to as group-level assessments, GLAs) with various stakeholders in the two neighborhoods and interviews with local parents, teachers, and administrators. The information collected from the GLAs and interviews was to be used to inform door-to-door surveys and follow-up "bright spot" household interviews. The result of the proposed research activities would include a list of assets and potential assets on multiple levels and the identification of barriers that were prohibiting access to these assets.

CAKE was created as a CAB–co-researcher hybrid model. Understanding what has worked well in previous CABs and co-researcher community-engaged projects provides us with a guide for evaluating our efforts. The rest of this section describes CAKE processes in the context of the three key domains for CABs: formation, operation, and maintenance.

The Formation of CAKE: CAB–Co-Researcher Hybrid Model

The first important step of the formation process is identifying and recruiting the right members. Community CAKE members were recruited using existing connections within the neighborhoods. To create the diverse team that was needed, IR leaders settled on identifying members that had some connection to Carthage or Roselawn and met one of three main criteria: (1) knowledge of early childhood education, (2) connections to Hispanic immigrant populations, or (3) community connections/active in the community. In addition, IR leaders sought representation from the various ethnic and racial groups in the neighborhoods (white, black, Hispanic). The initial goal was to have between five and ten community CAKE members, and we initially invited five members. Three additional members were added based on feedback from the initial five members about who was missing.

In the formation phase of CABs, it is important that the purpose, roles, and function of the group are clearly stated. For example, if the role of community members is as advisors, they provide guidance and advice, but ultimately decisions are left to the academic researchers leading the project. IR leaders created CAKE using a CAB–co-researcher hybrid model, where the community CAKE members are equal partners with shared decision-making, but not all partners were expected to participate in all research activities. CAKE members were given clear responsibilities, with expectations of time, funding, and project outcomes. We established these at our first meeting, where IR leaders presented a brief introduction to the project, including project goals and core values for CAKE.

We feel very strongly that we have formed a cohesive, unified group that represents the early childhood interests in our neighborhoods. Our success in the formation stage was strengthened by the relationships that existed before the project started. IR leaders already had established connections within the neighborhoods that were leveraged to help create a strong team. A second formation process component that has helped contribute to our success is the creation of a name and brand for ourselves. Before CAKE became CAKE, we did not have an identity, so one of the first things we did was to create one together as a group. We worked together at our second and third monthly meetings to create a name that was catchy and represented our values. We worked with a professional designer using a participatory design approach to develop a logo. After that, every communication representing our team was branded with the CAKE logo. We made T-shirts for every team member and tote bags to distribute to every research participant with our logo so we could become a recognizable entity in the community.

While we did a good job of establishing CAKE's purpose and roles, we could have been clearer about future roles related to research activities.

All CAKE members are involved with research activities at monthly meetings, but some members are paid to take a more active role in some of the research activities (e.g., administering surveys). This has caused some confusion and anxiety among other members, who assumed that all members would be taking part in all activities. A second weakness is related to the composition of the team. In hindsight, we realized we should have prioritized having a leader from each of the neighborhood councils as part of the team. While we have worked with the councils and have been engaged with them to some extent, we have lacked a consistent connection. We are working to improve this by designating specific CAKE community members to serve as liaisons, attending every community council meeting, reporting back to CAKE, and representing CAKE interests at community council meetings. It also would have been useful to attempt to recruit a policy member. While we have been engaged with key policy stakeholders—for example, Cincinnati Preschool Promise—it would have been helpful to have someone at a policy level as part of the team. We have worked to improve this by inviting CPP leadership to come speak to our group and having one CAKE member become part of CPP committees.

CAKE Operations: Establishing Core Values

Operation processes of CABs include establishing clear operating principles, leadership, and decision-making structure, and defining the logistical operations. Beginning with an understanding of the challenges of working across disciplines, particularly as it pertains to working within a community-based participatory research orientation, one of the first tasks we accomplished as IR leaders was to establish core values: (1) shared decision-making, (2) asset focused, and (3) real-world change. These values are what IR leaders each deemed most necessary when it came to the outcomes we want to achieve through our project. During our first meeting with the full CAKE leadership team, we discussed these values as a cohesive group and came to the unanimous decision to adopt them as CAKE's guiding values.

The core values of our group guide every aspect of our work together. This ensures that our research focuses on issues that are prioritized by the community and maximizes the potential for real-world impact. The first of these values is shared decision-making, of which trust and transparency are important components. We understand that power dynamics and positionality can create tension in partnerships and wanted to establish up front that the expertise of all partners is equally important to the success of the project. Every aspect of research design is overseen by the eleven-member CAKE leadership team, who collectively make decisions about activities throughout the research process. Our second value is that we are asset-focused. Communities are weary of traditional needs-based research approaches, with researchers often coming in and telling them what is wrong. Asset-based approaches offer a more positive way of identifying and enhancing community and household assets that exist within communities. For example, an asset that exists in our communities are churches, which serve as community hubs, led by trusted pastors doing activism work toward social justice in our city. We aim to work with and in these churches to improve early childhood wellness. Our final value is real-world change. Because the CAKE leadership team came together with the motivation of real-world change at the onset, it helped alleviate initial concerns of CAKE members that this would not be a traditional research project. Instead of the traditional transactional relationship between community and researchers, the research team would include community members as co-researchers and equal partners, where real-world change—not publications—is identified as the primary outcome. At every CAKE leadership team meeting, we check in on our progress toward real-world change, and CAKE members have held the group accountable when they have felt that we have been "spinning our wheels."

We have put our core values into practice in many activities, but the best example is the process we use for CAKE leadership team monthly lunch meetings. We build on assets in the community by always holding our meetings in one of our two neighborhoods, usually at New Prospect Baptist Church in Roselawn (where Morris serves as a community organizer) or Carthage Christian Church (where one of our CAKE members is the pastor). We demonstrate our value for having all CAKE leadership team members be equal partners by paying community members for their time and providing them with lunch. The IR leaders collectively set the agenda, and one of the three leads the meetings. We emphasize the importance of building relationships by using the first ten to fifteen minutes for informal conversation, catching up, and getting food. One of the IR leaders then introduces the meeting agenda and begins with any updates from the previous month (e.g., talking about past community events, reminders regarding upcoming events, progress on research activities). For most months there is one key theme for the meeting, which takes up the majority of meeting time. For example, some meetings are focused on planning research activities, reviewing research results, and discussing ways to connect with key stakeholders. We keep our focus on real-world change by concluding each meeting with a review of actions needed to be taken (e.g., Topmiller to follow up with policy stakeholders; Morris to work with one community member on planning parent meetings).

Research activities were initially planned by IR leaders, then presented and discussed at monthly meetings. While all CAKE members were involved with research activities through monthly meetings and email communication, participation levels in research activities varied significantly. For example, several members participated in our first research activity, group-level assessments (GLAs). We conducted four participatory focus groups (GLAs) with preschool provider union members, an African American Baptist church, a Hispanic Catholic church, and neighborhood council members. Overall, about one hundred people participated in the GLAs, where goals were to identify community assets and needs for early child wellness in Carthage and Roselawn. The GLAs served not only as data-gathering sessions but also as a strategy for achieving our aim of creating a network of engaged community members ready for future action toward early child health research. A GLA is a participatory and qualitative large group (fifteen to sixty participants) method in which valid data is generated and analyzed through an interactive and collaborative process (Vaughn et al. 2011; Vaughn and Lohmueller 1998). In contrast to other traditional qualitative methods, the GLA is not researcher-driven. Rather, various levels and statuses of academic and community stakeholders actively engage in data generation, participatory qualitative analysis, and action planning during the GLA process. Unlike more traditional focus group methods, GLAs allow "participants" an active voice and build capacity for shared decision-making between community and academic partners. Clear themes emerged across the GLAs, as participants identified a lack of access to community places and activities for young kids; the need for high-quality education programs that emphasized social, mental, and emotional health; and the desire for more parenting resources to support young parents.

All CAKE members took part in a monthly meeting dedicated to analyzing the results of the GLAs and took part in a pass-the-buck exercise to
transform the data into specific questions that could be included in future
interviews or surveys. The pass-the-buck exercise involved breaking into
three small groups and exploring the results of the GLAs on multiple
levels—household, school, and neighborhood. Each group took turns
reviewing the GLA results and adding questions on each of the levels.
The final result was a list of potential survey or interview questions for
each of the levels that have been used in later stages of the research. In
addition to the GLA research activities, all CAKE members reviewed and
gave feedback on interview and survey questions for neighborhood preschool providers and parents. Two CAKE members—with expertise in
the area—were asked to review the surveys one-on-one with IR leaders,
were trained in survey research methods, and took part in research ethics
training so they could administer surveys within their community.

The best example for demonstrating the power of having shared decision-making as a core value involves CAKE deciding to change research
plans and activities. Our initial grant proposal included conducting about
three hundred household surveys and follow-up "bright spot" household
interviews with about ten households. After reviewing the plans and
results from the GLAs, the group decided that the door-to-door surveys
would not be an appropriate use of resources. While the door-to-door
surveys and follow-up interviews had the potential to be an innovative
research project, there was no clear link between surveys and improvements in early childhood wellness in our neighborhoods. As a group,
CAKE decided to change the research plan to conduct surveys with all
early childhood providers in our neighborhoods and work through providers to reach out to parents.

CAKE members have also been involved with other neighborhood projects that are not directly related to the research plan or activities. For example, CAKE has been closely involved with the development of a new community recreation center in the neighborhood. IR leaders helped plan a small asset-mapping project with a group of AmeriCorps members in Carthage and worked with neighborhood leaders on a grant focused on increasing urban agricultural capacity in the neighborhood. Also, CAKE organized a small group of parents around understanding parent needs related to Cincinnati Preschool Promise and set up meetings with board members from Cincinnati Public Schools.

Maintenance of CAKE: Self-Evaluation and Plans for Sustainability

Two key components of maintenance processes for CABs include evaluation and sustainability. CAKE completed a self-evaluation at the midway point of our project, which provided important insights about improving as we move forward. We learned that CAKE members were particularly happy with the shared decision-making structure and appreciated the opportunities to collaborate with other neighborhood stakeholders, while also noting networking as one of the most important aspects of the project. We also found that our community co-researchers shared similar thoughts to IR leaders and were anxious to develop tangible, observable outputs. In the words of one leadership team member, "We have developed the container, now it's time to fill it up." We decided to reconnect with Cincinnati Preschool Promise to identify specific, tangible ways we could improve preschool access for youth children in our neighborhoods.

Our primary focus for sustainability is building capacity within Roselawn and Carthage for community engagement, awareness, and action. By funding community members on the CAKE leadership team, we hope to not only give them the ability to invest time and energy into our project but also to showcase the power of their perspectives to the larger Cincinnati community. One of the weaknesses of our project, however, has been a lack of a clear sustainability plan. Our initial proposal described a vague plan for sustainability built on the idea that we would be creating a network of advocates. However, we never specified a clear mechanism for sustaining our efforts. In our last year of Robert Wood Johnson Foundation (RJWF) funding, we are working to develop a concrete plan for sustainability that builds on CAKE connections to put action items into place. For example, CAKE is responding to the community-prioritized need for space and activities in the neighborhood where families can engage with each other and the larger community. To pursue an idea generated in CAKE leadership team meetings, we are partnering with local churches and faculty members from the University of Cincinnati College-Conservatory of Music to apply for funding to bring youth music programs to our neighborhoods. CAKE members have also strengthened ties with the nonprofit organizing universal preschool in our area, joining committees and workgroups to ensure that our communities' voices are heard when policies are made.

Conclusion: Reflections on Creating a Successful Community-Academic Partnership

Our project makes important contributions to interdisciplinary community-based scholarship by providing a blueprint process for engaging diverse community stakeholders into research efforts that result in real-world impact. Funding opportunities from the National Institutes of Health are increasingly requiring community-engaged approaches to interventions, leaving many traditional academic medicine investigators wondering how to meaningfully engage the community in their research efforts. Our project engaged eight community representatives who are responsible for sharing decision-making with researchers on each step of the research process. Our CAB–co-researcher hybrid model can be replicated by other community-engaged researchers who want to ensure that their research prioritizes community needs. Our experience with CAKE has provided us with important lessons about the formation, operation, and sustainability of community-academic partnerships.

Formation Lessons

In reflecting on the formation of our CAB–co-researcher hybrid leadership team, we identified several strategies and activities that were especially effective. We were able to take advantage of existing neighborhood connections and use an iterative recruitment process to bring together community leaders with diverse areas of expertise. We were purposeful in choosing the team to ensure we had lived experience expertise at the table, including parents of preschool-age children, churches in our two neighborhoods, and Latino-immigrant-serving organizations. We also were careful to recruit community leaders in early childhood education to ensure our work would represent what is really happening in preschools in our neighborhoods. We were extremely fortunate to have funding to pay CAKE leaders and to use a participatory design process to create a name and logo that allowed us to communicate our purpose and values to the larger community.

We also learned lessons that will inform the formation stage in future projects. First, we started our project with a broad focus on improving early childhood wellness in Carthage and Roselawn. We purposely kept our focus broad because we wanted to let the communities' voices

shape our research questions. We were hoping to identify a clear target
for intervention that was consistently prioritized across the many stakeholders we engaged, but one specific target did not emerge. Despite our
best intentions, the broad focus made it difficult to shape our narrative
and find our place in the larger system of providers and advocates for
early childhood services in Cincinnati. Second, we invited CAKE leaders
to the table and created an infrastructure that paid them for attending
meetings. We expected CAKE members to work outside of meetings
as co-researchers, but we did not lay out specific expectations or goals.
As a result, members were unclear what to do outside of our meetings
and began to feel uncertain about our accomplishments. In the future
we would collaboratively create roles and expectations for each CAKE
member and check in monthly on each person's goal progress.

Operation Lessons

In reflecting on the operation strategies that were most effective, we
believe our consistent emphasis on core values has been the most fruitful.
Our core values—that work be shared decision-making, asset-based, and
action-oriented—appear on each printed agenda. Our focus on these core
values from the formation of our team continues to inform the way we
operate even two years into the project. The most significant sign that
our core values were reflected in our operations was our collective decision to change the course of the research design we originally proposed
to our funders. We had originally planned a household survey across our
two neighborhoods that would identify "bright spots" in early childhood
wellness that could be replicated. After completing the group-level assessments, the CAKE team decided that the household surveys would not
be the most efficient or productive way to use resources and would not

provide a clear enough path toward action. Therefore, we changed course to a research strategy that would more closely adhere to our core values. One of the key operational processes identified by Newman et al. (2011) was establishing a decision-making process. While it has been clear that community CAKE members share in decision-making, we never established a decision-making process, such as voting on important topics. Our process has been to talk about issues as a group, but we have not had any instances where we felt like we needed to vote. We believe that trust was a big part of this, as a community partner was one of the IR leaders. However, it is possible that some community CAKE members may not have voiced disagreement due to a lack of a mechanism for doing so. Although our process has allowed for excellent relationship-building and organic collaborative idea generation, we sometimes have a lack of clear action items and fuzzy follow-up after group meetings.

Another important operation process component that CAKE is working to improve is communication among members. While we have monthly meetings, there can be a lack of consistent communication. IR leaders have been discussing doing a weekly email update as a way to keep all members of the CAKE leadership team engaged in the project. Additionally, CAKE does not keep meeting minutes, which may be helpful for recapping meetings and reminding CAKE members about project activities and updates.

Maintenance Lessons

Several aspects of our operation have proven to be helpful in maintaining CAKE, including valuing relationship-building as part of our process and providing resources (e.g., food, funding) to make our meetings con-venient and content for all members. We have also made self-reflection and evaluation a priority. Our comprehensive self-evaluation, conducted through interviews administered by an outside person, highlighted our adherence to our core values and the importance of what our team is doing. Our self-evaluation also revealed areas that needed to be enhanced for successful maintenance. CAKE members were concerned about the lack of action, which helped us realize that our topic was too broad at the beginning, hindering our progress. We now realize that we have to balance relationship-building and action, and have been more diligent about keeping track of progress on action steps and discussing them at each meeting.

Like all grant-funded collaborations, CAKE's sustainability is dependent on identifying mechanisms to support our collaborations after funding from the Robert Wood Johnson Foundation ends. We plan to seek out funding to continue our work and to pilot an intervention that we collaboratively develop based on our community research. It is possible, however, that CAKE will not exist in the same form after RWJF funding ends, but instead will result in CAKE members pursuing partnerships with other agencies in Cincinnati that were facilitated and grown during our funding period. For example, individual CAKE members are applying for grants with community agencies we have connected with as a group. Individual CAKE members are joining boards and committees to represent CAKE interests and will likely grow in their capacities with these groups long after CAKE funding ends. Even without a clear mechanism to sustain our group, we have planted our seeds throughout the city to ensure our work continues to support the growth of happy, healthy kids in Carthage and Roselawn.

References

Allen, J., G. W. Mohatt, K. L. Hazel, M. Rasmus, L. R. Thomas, and S. Lindley. 2006. "The Tools to Understand: Community as Co-Researcher on Culture Specific Protective Factors for Alaska Natives." *Journal of Prevention and Intervention in the Community* 32 (1): 41–59.

Andrews, J. O., G. Bentley, S. Crawford, L. Pretlow, and M. S. Tingen. 2007. "Using Community-Based Participatory Research to Develop a Culturally Sensitive Smoking Cessation Intervention with Public Housing Neighborhoods." *Ethnicity & Disease* 17 (2): 331–37.

Brookes, B. 2006. "Introduction to History, Health, and Hybridity." *Health and History* 8 (1): 1–3.

Dankwa-Mullan, I., and E. J. Pérez-Stable. 2016. "Addressing Health Disparities Is a Place-Based Issue." *American Journal of Public Health* 106 (4): 637–39.

Israel, B. A., A. J. Schulz, E. A. Parker, and A. B. Becker. 1998. "Review of Community-Based Research: Assessing Partnership Approaches to Improve Public Health." *Annual Review of Public Health* 19 (1): 173–202.

Jacquez, F. M., L. Vaughn, and G. Suarez-Cano. 2019. "Implementation of a Stress Intervention with Latino Immigrants in a Non-Traditional Migration City." *Journal of Immigrant and Minority Health* 21 (2): 372–82. doi: 10.1007/s10903-018-0732-7.

Morin, S. F., A. Maiorana, K. A. Koester, N. M. Sheon, and T. A. Richards. 2003. "Community Consultation in HIV Prevention Sesearch: A Study of Community Advisory Boards at 6 Research Sites." *Journal of Acquired Immune Deficiency Syndromes* 33 (4): 513–20.

National Center for Education Statistics (NCES). 2015–2016. "Hamilton County, Ohio. Public Schools [Data]." Elementary/Secondary Information System (ELSi). https://nces.ed.gov/Programs/Edge/ACSDashboard/4701590.

Newman, S., D. Maurer, A. Jackson, M. Saxon, R. Jones, and G. Reese. 2009. "Gathering the Evidence: Photovoice as a Tool for Disability Advocacy." *Progress in Community Health Partnerships* 3 (2): 139–44.

Newman, S. D., J. O. Andrews, G. S. Magwood, C. Jenkins, M. J. Cox, and D. C. Williamson. 2011. "Peer Reviewed: Community Advisory Boards in Community-Based Participatory Research: A Synthesis of Best Processes." *Preventing Chronic Disease* 8 (3): 1–12.

US Census Bureau. 2012–2016. "Cincinnati City, Ohio; DP03 Selected Economic Characteristics [Data]." 2014 American Community Survey 5-Year Estimates.

Vaughn, L. M., and M. Lohmueller. 1998. "Using the Group-Level Assessment in a Support Group Setting." *Organization Development Journal* 16 (1): 99–105.

Vaughn, L. M., F. Jacquez, J. Zhao, and M. Lang. 2011. "Partnering with Students to Explore the Health Needs of an Ethnically Diverse, Low-Resource School: An Innovative Large Group Assessment Approach." *Family & Community Health* 34 (1): 72–84.

Vaughn, L. M., C. Whetstone, A. Boards, M. D. Busch, M. Magnusson, and S. Määttä. 2018. "Partnering with Insiders: A Review of Peer Models across Community-Engaged Research, Education and Social Care." *Health & Social Care in the Community* 26 (6): 769–86.

Chapter 4

Finding Our Way as a Cross-Systems Team

Lessons Learned from an Interdisciplinary Research Team

Karen Ruprecht
ICF International, Inc.

Angela Tomlin
Indiana University School of Medicine

Shoshanna Spector
Faith in Indiana

Chapter Context

Our team members brought backgrounds in early childhood education and early childhood mental health. These included supporting the parent-child relationship when parents are incarcerated and community leadership and advocacy around the issue of mass incarceration. The state of Indiana has a high level of incarceration; however, some programs, such as Faith in Indiana, have had success in working with local congregations to both raise awareness to the problem and create meaningful change. We wanted to take the idea that incarceration affects the whole family, especially young children, who have not been well represented in the research, and consider if high-quality early care could support these children and families. Our chapter discusses our experiences in overcoming differences and learning to work cooperatively to achieve shared interests.

Our research sought to learn how many young children (three to six years years old) in Indiana experience parental incarceration. We collected surveys from community members and 666 preschool providers (nearly 20 percent of all preschool providers in Indiana) about their experiences with children who have an incarcerated parent. From those surveyed, it was determined that approximately 1,500 preschool children, or 6 percent, have a parent who is incarcerated. National surveys indicate that 10 percent of children from the ages of birth to five years have lived with a parent who has been incarcerated in their lifetime. We next conducted focus groups to learn from affected community members and early care workers about their lived experiences with children who have incarcerated parents. Much information was gleaned from these focus groups—how children and parents responded to separation due to incarceration; the influence of incarceration on parental decisions, such as whether to send their child to preschool; whether to inform the preschool about the incarceration; and whether the parents viewed preschool as beneficial to their children. We also learned how informed providers were about family experiences, how they responded to the children in their care who had an incarcerated parent, and what they need to best serve these children and families.

Our project goals and methods changed over time as we learned more about the work and each other. At times we struggled to work together due to differences that included understanding of research, familiarity with community organization, and work styles. Our chapter discusses our team's development across the project and provides key takeaways from each stage of our team process. An important overarching theme is the need to recognize and honor the amount of upfront work, planning, and time it takes to form relationships necessary to progress the work. A second important takeaway is that change is always happening in the team, requiring flexibility and a certain amount of forgiveness. As our team is completing our project, we continue to realize that we can still learn from each other.

Introduction

Interdisciplinary teams are increasingly common as more researchers address complex community issues that require expertise in more than one discipline (Boaz, Biri, and McKevitt 2016). Issues such as addressing health inequities, implementation science, and translational science all are areas ripe for interdisciplinary research (Tebes and Thai 2018). Building a research team composed of university researchers and community advocates requires a different and unique approach to teaming and a different research framework than the typical university structure for conducting research. In the conventional academic setting, research occurs in a hierarchical organization. Most university-based research projects originate from a department or lab of a principal investigator who is the lead in charge of the research design. The work is often carried out with a team of junior researchers and graduate students, who help recruit the study participants, perform data collection duties, analyze data, and perform the initial analyses. Often—if not always—study results are not shared with the study participants directly. Recognition and dissemination may be shared within the research team, but typically community members that participate in the research do not receive credit or recognition for their participation in the research (Thebes and Thai 2018).

The ways traditional academic researchers and community-based organizations view, engage in, and use data derived from research are often very different. These differences may stem from divergent training backgrounds and work setting expectations, which create equally divergent understandings about the purpose of the work and the data it generates. For example, university-based researchers often view research as contributing discrete pieces of information to a knowledge base; they may not see a need for the work to have an immediate practical application.

Often academically situated researchers are pressured to share their results with other professionals in ways that lead to academic advancement—for example, conference presentations and publishing in peer-reviewed journals. In contrast, community-based organizations may view research as useful primarily to the extent that the results directly and immediately impact the populations they serve. For example, a community-based organization may use data to support or confirm their current or future program plans; identify trends in demographics, characteristics, issues, or outcomes that support the overall aims of their programs; or influence public policy. As a result, those from community-based organizations may be eager to disseminate findings broadly to a variety of audiences, often framing the research findings in bold terms that include a call to action. In contrast, researchers tend to be significantly more cautious in discussing the implications and limitations of data. These types of differences in thinking about the meaning and purpose of research results can set the stage for different and conflicting goals that may stress cross-system team partnerships. With good planning and communication, however, research teams and community advocates can generate work that results in more innovation, greater learning across systems, meaningful contributions to science and to public policy and program improvement.

This chapter focuses on the experience working as a new team of professionals from academic and community-based institutions to conduct research on access to high-quality pre-kindergarten (pre-k) education for children whose caregivers experienced incarceration. We detail our challenges, successes, and lessons learned throughout the process of team development, research planning and implementation, and our beginning forays into dissemination. The discussion includes a frank assessment of the hits and misses as we worked toward team integration. The team's challenges in learning each other's communication styles are also discussed, highlighting the often overlooked but very powerful reasons why communication is integral to team success. Finally we discuss efforts to become more aligned and effective as a team from the perspective of the growing recognition that the process of building a research team may be just as important as the outcome of the research (Tebes and Thai 2018).

Identifying A Model to Reflect on Team Processes

When research teams come together and represent different interests, having tools or processes to help guide the research and communication process are useful. Some research collaborations have developed a field guide to help the team develop a shared vision and goals, discuss recognition and dissemination efforts, and help guide communication efforts, including ways to build trust and address conflict within the team (Bennett, Gadlin, and Levine-Finley 2010). The use of a field guide or similar tools helps interdisciplinary research teams come to a shared understanding of the research goals, develop team cohesion, and lay out common expectations among members of the group.

For the current retrospective analysis of our team processes, we loosely adapted an integrated example and framework of participatory team science to help organize reflections about the team experience (Hall et al. 2012). This framework divides team research into four phases with associated tasks or activities. Although the team had experiences in all of the described tasks, the team did not go through the experiences in the linear sequence described, so our personal process differs from Hall's model in a few ways. Most notably, we revisited the processes related to communication, role assignment, and defining the research question several times. Additionally, we describe both internal factors about team member attributes—such as personality and training background—and external factors—including the fellowship that brought the team together, our individual work environments, and overall factors that we see as affecting the group process. In the following sections we refer to the four phases and associated tasks as we outline our team progress, including missteps, the repairs made, and the lessons learned.

- *Becoming a team*—development phase: Team members define the problem, develop a shared understanding and model to study the problem, and establish a team identity.
- *Preparing to do the work*—conceptualization phase: Team members identify research questions and design, establish communication practices within the team, and specify team roles and responsibilities.
- *Doing and learning from the work*—implementation phase: Team members conduct the research, coordinate work and make adjustments as needed, manage conflict, and integrate what is learned from the research process.
- *Sharing what was learned and taking next steps*—translation phase: Team members apply what has been learned to address challenges and develop relevant partnerships for dissemination and translation.

Getting Started: The Interdisciplinary Team

The team came together as a result of a fellowship opportunity offered by the Robert Wood Johnson Foundation (RWJF). In 2016 the RWJF initiated the Interdisciplinary Research Leaders (IRL) fellowship as part of their efforts to build a fulture of health through the development of teams that partnered community advocates and researchers to address critical questions around health equity in their communities. The teams received financial support, online and face-to-face training, mentorship, and other experiences intended to equip them to collectively conduct research that leads to outcomes with direct relevance to critical community issues. Our team was one of fifteen teams selected in the inaugural cohort, and focused on early childhood education.

Prior to being selected to participate in the program, team members had no shared history of working or collaborating together. The initial creation of the team happened quickly and through a snowball approach. First the community advocate learned of the fellowship opportunity and realized the potential to marry the organization's interest in reducing mass incarceration with efforts in the state to expand and promote state-funded pre-k. The community advocate reached out to state leaders working to advance pre-k expansion, which led to a connection with a childcare researcher at a statewide early learning organization. The childcare researcher invited a specialist in infant and early childhood mental health who had experience working with incarcerated mothers to join the team.

The team's strengths included members who are highly experienced, are well connected, and demonstrated leadership capacity. All three members were excited about the fellowship opportunity and eager to partner; however, as a result of the way the team was assembled, none of the members knew the others or their work well. Furthermore, due to a short timeline to develop and submit an application, team members managed only some brief face-to-face and phone contacts in pairs prior to submitting the proposal; the entire three-member team never met in person prior to submission. This circumstance meant that each member contributed to the proposal and addressed their specific area of expertise in isolation, without having the opportunity to come together and create a shared vision that combined the community challenge of mass incarceration and access to high-quality education for children of incarcerated parents. The team's communication was disjointed from the beginning, and over time this affected all aspects of the team's progress.

In the first few months of the research and fellowship program, the team struggled to figure out how to work together, and there were many miscommunications. It is important to point out that the fellowship program itself was also under construction, as the group was the inaugural cohort. The program's leadership was transparent in stating they were "building the plane while flying it," so there was a parallel process of the leadership group's development that happened along with the team's process. There was genuine excitement about the opportunity and the potential of the work. Despite this excitement about a new collaborative and interdisciplinary process, the team did not take time to build a communication infrastructure up front and had to work on this throughout the rest of the experience.

Becoming a Team: Development Phase

During the development phase, research partners and community advocates form a team based on a mutual interest in addressing a shared problem (Tebes and Thai 2018). It is recommended that teams spend time in this period to identify goals and to build trust and mutual respect among all members. These steps are meant to form a frame that will allow the team to withstand expected conflicts and setbacks. In this section, we focus on our challenges in becoming a team and the communication deficits underlying our difficulties. Although a significant amount of information, training modules, and tools were made available as part of our participation in the fellowship program, we were not able to use these effectively at the time.

As discussed earlier, the team came together quickly, and there was no time for formal team-building activities during the application process.

This is not a surprise, as members' numerous personal and professional commitments is a common barrier to teams seeking to improve collaboration (Drahota et al. 2016). Even after the team was formalized, time was not devoted to clearly identify their mission and goals, to build trust, and to establish a team identity. The only "team" part that existed at the beginning of the collaboration was the fact that a fellowship had been awarded to three individuals with significant and complementary skill and expertise in their respective disciplines.

As the team began to form, some steps were either rushed and did not feel genuine, or were skipped altogether. For example, in one of the first meetings, the community advocate encouraged the researchers to share their personal stories about who they were and what brought them to their work. While this is a common community-organizing activity, it is not typical for researchers to share personal information in a professional setting. This expectation to share personal information so early on was not well understood by the research partners and felt forced and uncomfortable, as trust was not yet established. This episode may reflect the different expectations that the community and research partners brought into the team-building experience.

A second barrier to team building was the richness of the training offered by fellowship. Experiencing tension with pressure to complete project tasks versus developing the team is common. As described by Drahota et al., "Where to put one's energy is a constant dilemma" (2016, 190). Each team member had the opportunity to participate in online courses, complete team-building exercises, participate in two face-to-face meetings requiring out-of-state travel, and contribute to the team's research proposal in the first four months of the fellowship program. Therefore, personal education opportunities, required activities, and team building competed for available time. In addition, much of this information was new to the team members. Taking in new concepts can create disruption and requires time to integrate (Thebes and Thai 2018).

The diversity of the team members in terms of skill sets and work styles was another factor that had positive and negative aspects. Team members had some surface similarities (gender, race), but were diverse in deep-level ways related to life experience, knowledge, and skills (Harrison, Price, and Bell 1998). Opportunity existed in the diversity of the team members' backgrounds, which could allow for true innovation (Edmondson and Harvey 2017). At the same time, this diversity in backgrounds created a lack of shared understanding between team members about each other, and the overall project goals were another factor that contributed to the communication problems that slowed and even derailed the work.

A final barrier to the development of a team identity was poor agreement about the actual team member composition. From the outset of the process, the community-based team member conceptualized the team more broadly than the research members, who focused on the three individuals who applied and were selected for the fellowship. The community-based partner was much more expansive and envisioned the team as including those three fellows, the project manager, other assistants, and many community members who could contribute in a variety of ways. This broader team was much more diverse than the three fellowship members. Although the larger team possessed many advantages—for example, firsthand knowledge of community stakeholders, the potential for wider knowledge and skill sets to draw on, more hands to complete work—it was also more unwieldy to coordinate and created more opportunities for miscommunication, which had to be managed.

Lessons Learned: Development Phase

The main lesson learned from the experience during this phase can be summarized as *do the team-building activities!* The team experienced one of the most common barriers to teamwork—time pressure. In retrospect it was clear that taking the time to get to know each other and to discuss in detail the work and beliefs would have created a stronger team and avoided problems down the road.

The second lesson is *no, really, do the team-building activities!* Through the fellowship program, the team had access to an online course and tools related to team process. The team was split regarding the value and necessity of doing these activities. The community advocate expressed confidence that the team had discussed these topics sufficiently during an initial meeting and so did not want to expend additional effort on the process. Although they felt pressure to move through the process and get to the research piece, the research team wanted to complete the assignments. Frankly this preference was partly due to wanting to improve the team process but also because the academically oriented researchers valued completing "assignments" and realized the value of reflecting on the team process. In the end, the team completed the communication contract, which accurately pointed out the problem areas. Since the process was completed to fulfill a requirement rather than to think about how individual communication styles impacted the team process, the findings were not used to improve team communication.

A final lesson from this experience is *build on team member's strengths.* The team's strength was and continues to be the members' ability to complete tasks independently and together. This allowed the team to make progress and accomplish tasks despite the challenges that were experienced related to team identity and communication. The team experienced success and fulfilled requirements, but it was harder than it had to be. As described in the next section, the team's initial failure to come together created an unstable foundation, slowing the work.

Preparing to Do the Work: Conceptualization Phase

During the conceptualization phase, the team develops research questions and research design in partnership with community members, setting the stage to do the work in the next phase. Key underlying activities to success in this phase are establishing communication structures and practices and identifying roles and responsibilities within the team (Hall et al. 2012). Because the developmental tasks were not fully addressed during phase one, entering phase two found the team already out of sync. As mentioned earlier, the compressed time frame to complete a required grant proposal to access research funds and the plethora of opportunities within the fellowship continued to compete for time and attention. In addition to the lingering struggle to clarify the team's identity, there were issues related to achieving a unified voice regarding the purpose of the research and determining who would do what parts of the work. The intensity of the process also revealed many differences about the team members' preferred work styles and flow.

The original research questions were: How many preschool children in the state have an incarcerated parent? What are the barriers and challenges to accessing high-quality preschool for those children? Is high-quality preschool a buffer to the stresses of experiencing parental incarceration? Differences in understanding the primary focus of the research became apparent when team members talked about the research project to community groups and other fellowship cohort teams. Specifically, the researchers tended to describe the project in a narrow way, focusing on the aspect of the effects of incarceration on children, whereas the community advocate spoke in broader terms of the importance of reducing mass incarceration and rarely invoked the research questions regarding preschool. In short, the team was divided as to the main thrust of the work—the problem of mass incarceration versus the problem of the need for access to pre-k for children with parents who have experienced incarceration. As a result, both completing the research proposal and preparing to move into the implementation phase became more difficult because of the lack of a shared understanding of the problem from both the advocate and researchers' viewpoints.

Decision-making about team members' roles and responsibilities is also important in this phase. It is common for each group to enter the team process with different ideas about role functions and priorities (Edmondson and Harvey 2017). The previous omission of a team-building process meant that it took longer to get to know each other as individuals—for example, what we know, what we do, and who we are—which is a prerequisite to understanding how each person would function as part of the team. In general, team members need social interactions over time to promote trust, collaboration, and team identity. These social interactions can produce emotional, cognitive, and motivational states within individual team members, which, in turn, promote knowledge integration within the team (Salas, Fiore, and Letsky 2013; Salazar et al. 2012). Knowledge integration among and across disciplines is valuable because it allows team members to build on their individual and combined competencies to explore different perspectives and ask deeper questions than is possible through one discipline (Bozeman and Boardman 2014). Because the team was delayed in getting to know each member on an individual level, it was not possible to know how each would be within the team, making it difficult to feel confident in assigning team roles.

The team discovered there were different expectations related to the specific activities that needed to be accomplished and who would do them. For some team members, participation in the fellowship meant taking part in all available opportunities—for example, leadership training, meetings, and the research—but others preferred to limit their participation to selected activities. The community-based team member voiced the expectation that a project manager would serve as the point person from the community organization and fulfill the duties as a main liaison with the researchers. The other team members were aware that hiring a project director was planned but understood the role to be limited to supporting the research. These team members assumed that the other fellowship responsibilities would continue to fall to the original recipients. Over time the researchers recognized the value of this broader approach, but initially the difference in viewpoints led to friction.

Differences in the team members' work styles interfered with the effectiveness of the team and, at times, disrupted trust. Some worked in spurts—some slowly over time. There were several occasions when the community team member made decisions and communicated information to outsiders prior to discussion within the team. This was upsetting for the research team members and required several discussions to resolve. For example, the community advocate requested an extension to the deadline to submit the grant proposal without the researchers' knowledge. The community-based team member was comfortable seeking extensions in such situations, whereas the researchers, used to federal agencies with strict deadlines, were reluctant to request such accommodations.

The workflow and work style challenges were exacerbated by ongoing differences in preferred communication methods and styles. For example, after the project manager joined the group, she began participating in weekly research calls, ensuring that relevant information from the community organization was known to all. The other members of the team assumed that the project manager would also relay research planning discussions to the other community team members. However, it soon became apparent that the information discussed in the research calls was not consistently shared with the community advocate. After some reflection, the researchers realized that the community team members often used text messaging to communicate a wide range of information; the research team members tended to use email, including sending minutes of each team meeting. The research members were unaware that email communications were not always read by community team members, and the community team members were not aware that these messages contained important details. Thus, important research communications were not conveyed.

Lessons Learned: Conceptualization Phase

Echoing the lessons from the development phase, the first lesson in the conceptualization phase was *talk to each other regularly*. The failure to complete the team-development process continued to interfere with the work in the conceptualization phase. A team that did not fully form and that did not take time to come to an agreement regarding communication could be expected to struggle to come to an agreement about other important functions, such as team roles. In response, regular weekly research calls between the researchers and the project manager served a number of purposes, including creating familiarity and relationship needed for trust, maintaining lines of communication, and creating timelines and accountability to move ahead with accomplishing tasks. This adjustment also helped the team plan ahead and account for the differing work styles and preferences. Team members still had different work-flows but were open about these differences and divided tasks in ways that allowed the team to make progress in completing research activities. The regular calls also gave the team members time to get to know each other better.

Despite that success, establishing regular meeting time alone was not enough to avoid some of the pitfalls that the communication problems brought. The second lesson in this phase was *be aware of differences in workplace culture and terminology*. For the team, this included continuing problems with communication (email versus text) discussed earlier; there were other instances of team members not receiving communications. Differences in workplace culture were also evident. For example, the project manager arranged for local university undergraduate students to help with data entry of a community survey. As one of the researchers started to lead the students through the process, she introduced herself using her title instead of her first name. Later the project manager explained that this title surprised her and that she had never thought about the researcher in that way. The same researcher later noticed the project manager hesitating when about to introduce her to a community group. The researcher stepped in to introduce herself, this time without her title. In this group, the researcher wanted to be seen as a person who was there to learn from the community members' firsthand knowledge. These two experiences were useful ways to think about how researchers present themselves in different settings when working across systems and the meaning of different terms and practices in different settings. For example, presenting oneself as more relatable can be more important in informal than in formal settings; setting the appropriate tone is critical.

As mentioned earlier, the results of a communication assessment suggested that the team should address this area to be successful in the research project. The third lesson from this part of the team development is *vary the ways to learn about each other*. A range of team-building activities related to team process was recommended, one of which was to create a visual representation of team development based on the metaphor of a river. After initial reluctance by some members to do the "art project," the team used paper and markers to create a mural. The mural included a series of images depicting the team stepping off the dock; riding in a boat on relatively calm seas that changed into a rough sea; and obstacles (waves, rocks, and stormy clouds) representing personal and professional obligations that sometimes disrupted the team's ability to communicate with each other. The process of creating the mural and talking through challenges strengthened the team. Despite the acknowledgment of the somewhat stormy beginning, the team saw that the boat remained upright, and members remained committed to the cause. This gave hope that the completion of the research proposal—which was on the horizon—would be smoother.

Doing and Learning from the Work: Implementation Phase

According to Hall et al. (2012), the implementation phase of participatory team science is the phase where the research is conducted based on the group members' roles and responsibilities. This phase may require adjustments as the research project unfolds and requires the expertise of a range of individuals that might have connections to the community. Some important tasks during this phase included making revisions to the research design as needed, working through the university's process of approval for research, adjusting materials and methods to fit different participant groups, working together across systems as needed to purchase research related supplies, coordinating schedules to identify available times for focus groups held across the state, conducting the focus groups, and beginning the process of transcribing data in preparation for analysis.

Once the actual research activities began, it was easy for the research and community-based team members to fall into their typical roles. For example, the researchers focused on familiar tasks, including preparing the Institutional Review Board (IRB) and identifying the software that would be needed for data analysis. However, both research and community team members partnered for many of these activities. For example, the project manager and the other community team members led the process of identifying community members to help design the survey instruments, give recommendations about the wording of recruitment information, and help facilitate focus groups. The team expanded when one of the researchers added an assistant who was able to help with the project work. The assistant was able to coordinate scheduling focus group times and locations with community partners in the state, manage communication with focus group members, and assist with data entry.

The biggest adjustment made in this phase was in the method and design of the community research project. Initially the project proposed to survey and interview parents who had formerly been incarcerated or their partner had been incarcerated while they had a preschool-age child. The community advocate was very familiar with gathering data from large groups of people for community action, and this was not an unfamiliar task for her or her organization. It was common for the community organization to gather hundreds of surveys from the community, but the research approach was a bit different. The research called for a narrow subset of the population—people who had been formerly incarcerated or their partner—and then narrowed it further with the criteria that they had a preschool-age child when they or their partner were incarcerated. As the research team examined the surveys from the community, it became evident that this population was not being reached. Thus the research design was altered to include collecting survey data and conducting focus groups with preschool providers to determine what they knew about children in their care who had a parent that had been or was currently incarcerated. Their insight—coupled with that of the community members—has given the research a unique and deeper perspective into parent and provider experiences and has strengthened the research study.

Because of the unresolved issues with communication from the onset of the project, this portion of the research did not always go smoothly. On weekly research calls, the team members discussed shifting the focus and including preschool providers as part of the research design. Many of these conversations were documented in minutes or follow-up emails, which were sent to the team after the meeting. The revision of the research design was confirmed as a team and discussed with the fellowship leadership to ensure this shift was appropriate for the goals of the research. The researchers believed the information about shifting some of the research focus had been discussed and well documented with all the parties. However, it became evident when planning the community focus groups that the project manager did not have all the information about the change in the research plan. Through email communication, the researchers discovered that there were plans to invite twenty or more people to participate. The project manager, who was used to conducting community gatherings, thought the focus groups were similar to these community gatherings. The previous groundwork in developing trust and repairing misunderstanding was useful in addressing the miscommunication. The project manager reached out for clarification, and the research team members were quickly able to identify that the term *focus group* had not been defined. The discussion also revealed another kind of communication problem related to knowledge—the project manager was not familiar with the term *focus group* and so did not understand the researchers' use of that terminology meant a different process. The researchers did not realize the project manager misunderstood the term. A researcher named the problem, explained why the focus group had to be limited in size, and apologized for the poor communication. This was a nice repair to the team, and avoided a scenario of twenty people trying to share at one focus group.

Lessons Learned: Implementation Phase

As Hall et al. (2012) stated in their framework, interdisciplinary research teams should expect some changes to the research design and methods in this phase, and those changes should be welcomed as long as it strengthens the potential outcomes. Changing midcourse and including preschool providers as part of the research plan helped strengthen the research design and opened a new area of research for the team to con-sider in the future. However, poor communication almost derailed the team again when everyone felt in the loop about these changes. The first lesson learned in this segment is that smooth communication requires continual effort. The team needed to continually assess the effectiveness of its communication methods. As part of this assessment, the team found that terms such as *focus groups* conveyed different meanings between the researchers and the community advocates.

The data-collection schedule was tight and coincided with an import-ant time in the local election cycle. The team members working in the community organization were incredibly busy due to the increased number of activities needed to register voters. The community organization also moved during this time period, which is often stressful. The research partners also had extra commitments at this time of year—welcoming new clinical students, general teaching responsibilities, and grant-reporting deadlines. When under time pressure and other stressors, a common response is to fall back into old habits. Maintaining newly learned skills is much more difficult under such circumstances. Therefore, the second lesson in the implementation phase is *plans are nice, but they will be changed*. Because the team continued the regular meetings, there was deeper knowledge about each other's work and responsibilities. This allowed the team to support each other when making plans, schedules, and dividing up the work. Since the team was aware from the beginning of the year that autumn would be challenging for the community-based team members, the team was better able to develop a schedule that would work. The improved communication was also helpful when unexpected tasks or opportunities arose. Even though each team member had a lot of individual responsibilities, clear communication, flexibility, and a sense of shared responsibility to the team allowed the team to make progress.

The last lesson in this section relates to forgiveness when mistakes are made. It is well-known that teamwork is often complicated and messy. As the team got the chance to know each other better, we are less reactive to missteps from each other. The lesson here is *mistakes are learning opportunities*. The example of the misunderstanding over the term *focus group* is a prime example of how communication needs to be clear and the terms defined for all parties. The focus group experiences have had a few bumps as well. However, the team is learning from these challenges and each other.

Sharing What Was Learned and Taking Next Steps:
Translation Phase

In this final stage of the model, the team works to translate the findings of the research into real-world practice. While academic researchers typically wait until all data has been collected and analyzed before
publishing or sharing results, this phase of team science is focused on
translating the learning as it happens. Examples of activities during this
phase might include sharing emerging lessons learned from the research,
using emerging data to change practices in an organization or system, or
using data to help advocate for policy change.

The fellowship program included an emphasis on dissemination in
a broad sense. Multiple opportunities were offered for teams to learn
about dissemination, including webinars, face-to-face training, reading,
and mentorship. The intention was to build comfort in sharing data and
processes across multiple platforms and as the information is being gath-
ered. Learning to be comfortable with this approach was sometimes hard
for the research members of the team, who were used to waiting until
the final results have been written before sharing their project. While
certainly uncomfortable with this concept at the beginning of the fellowship, the researchers have embraced this concept wholeheartedly, and
have appreciated the support from the community organizer to frame
the context of the data. Each team member has delivered presentations at
state and national meetings regarding the team's research and has started
to share emerging findings from the survey and focus group data. The
community organizer and one of the researchers had long-standing relationships with local news organizations; therefore they were much more
comfortable and agile in giving interviews. The other researcher has less
experience in this arena; however, that team partner was able to gain skill

and experience in talking about the work through several interviews this last year.

Early in the process, the team did not have a good shared understanding of the focus of the work. As discussed earlier, the team struggled when the community team member's communication felt too slanted to incarceration in general rather than the effect on preschool children. However, with the increased attention and recognition of the importance of state-funded pre-k programs, the community advocates recognized the importance of this issue to their constituents. The issue of pre-k resonates with the community organization's stance (or motto) of "families first" and is front and center in the community team member's conversations and plans for legislative efforts. At a recent community focus group, there were multiple pieces of evidence that preschool is a key issue. For example, messaging about preschool is prominently included in the organization's posters, which were displayed in their meeting rooms. The focus group members recruited by the project manager and other community group staffers included formerly incarcerated individuals or individuals with a partner who was or who had been incarcerated; most were parents of preschool children. This was a relief to the researchers, who had been concerned about the community group's ability to identify and recruit this narrow population. One woman shared her knowledge of preschool with the group, including an explanation of the state's quality-rating-improvement system. A male participant thanked her for bringing the information to the group and talked about how important it was for the whole community to know about this system. Another man asked if anyone thought that their community was denied this information on purpose. Others discussed this possibility, making reference to the IRB materials that the researcher had shared.

It was exciting for the researcher to see and hear directly how information is being disseminated into the communities served. At the same time, it was surprising to hear participants wonder if the information had been withheld from them in some way. Although the researcher was well informed about the historical example of communities being mistreated in research, she had not directly heard this fear voiced. It is possible that the community-research partnership created a sense of trust that allowed the participant to voice this concern. This incident provides a clear example of how the research knowledge is being infused into community process; it also shows how the community understanding and response to information, in turn, can inform researchers.

Lessons Learned: Translation Phase

As this phase is still unfolding, the team is still learning lessons about how to translate community research to policymakers, advocates, and the research community. The biggest lesson learned so far in this phase is *try new things, even if it makes you uncomfortable*. Through this process, as the researchers have better understood dissemination more broadly, they have been able to discuss their understanding of findings as they emerge. The researchers are able to present research linking parental incarceration with the impact it has on young children without even presenting any data from the project. The researchers understand the value of bringing forward these ideas to legislators and the public over time in order to create interest, raise awareness, and build eagerness to learn more as the research proceeds. The second lesson the research team has learned in the translation phase is *learning goes both ways*. Researchers and communities have much to learn from each other. Through the relationships that have developed across systems, learning is possible. We continue to learn about the team process and know that we will take steps forward and back as we go. Those back-and-forth points of interactions across groups are where the magic happens.

Conclusion

Interdisciplinary research produces important knowledge that addresses community issues by bringing together academic partners and community advocates. This pairing of academics and community partners helps ensure research is meaningful and has utility for the communities it intends to help. As this experience highlighted, there is significant work the team should complete to function most effectively.

First, interdisciplinary teams should take time to develop a shared understanding of the issue the team wants to address. Initial discussions should focus on the purpose of the research so each member can clearly articulate the problem being studied. Team members should spend time getting to know each other as individuals and learn about each other's work history and organizational culture. This process helps establish a shared team identity and sets the stage for communication throughout the research process. Second, all team members should be involved in conceptualizing the research questions and the methods to establish the goals of the research. This helps clarify roles and responsibilities for each team member throughout the research process. When time is spent clarifying these roles, as the research unfolds and questions emerge, the team can be better positioned to address challenges and make course adjustments as needed. Throughout this entire process, frequent communication among team members is central to team success. We hope the honesty about our team's struggles to communicate effectively helps other interdisciplinary research teams as they engage in community-based research.

References

Bennett, L. M., H. Gadlin, and S. Levine-Finley. 2010. *Collaboration and Team Science: A Field Guide*. NIH publication no. 10-7660. Rockville, MD: National Institutes of Health.

Boaz, A., D. Biri, and C. McKevitt. 2016. "Rethinking the Relationship between Science and Society: Has There Been a Shift in Attitudes to Patient and Public Involvement and Public Engagement in Science in the United Kingdom?" *Health Expectations* 19 (3): 592–601. doi: 10.1111/hex.12295.

Bozeman, B., and C. Boardman. 2014. *Research Collaboration and Team Science: A State-of-the-Art Review and Agenda*. Basel, Switzerland: Springer Nature. doi: 10.1007/978-3-319-06468-0.

Drahota, A., R. Mezo, B. Brikho, M. Naaf, J. A. Estabillo, E. D. Gomez, and S. F. Vojnosk. 2016. "Community-Academic Partnerships: A Systematic Review of the State of the Literature and Recommendations for Future Research." *Milbank Quarterly* 94 (1): 163–214.

Edmondson, A. C., and J. F. Harvey. 2017. "Cross-Boundary Teaming for Innovation: Integrating Research on Teams and Knowledge in Organizations." *Human Resource Management Review* 28 (4): 347–60. doi: 10.1016/j.hrmr.2017.03.002.

Hall, K. L., A. L. Vogel, B. Stipelman, D. Stokols, G. Morgan, and S. Gehlert. 2012. "A Four-Phase Model of Transdisciplinary Team-Based Research: Goals, Team Processes, and Strategies." *Translational Behavioral Medicine* 2 (4): 415–30.

Harrison, D. A., and K. J. Klein. 2007. "What's the Difference? Diversity Constructs as Separation, Variety, or Disparity in Organizations." *Academy of Management Review* 32 (4): 1199–1228.

Harrison, D. A., K. H. Price, and K. P. Bell. 1998. "Beyond Relational Demography: Time and the Effects of Surface-and Deep-Level Diversity on Work Group Cohesion." *Academy of Management Journal* 41: 96–107.

Salas, E., S. M. Fiore, and M. P. Letsky. 2013. "Why Cross-Disciplinary Theories of Team Cognition?" In *Theories of Team Cognition: Crossdisciplinary Perspectives*, edited by E. Salas, S. M. Fiore, and M. P. Letsky, 41–63. New York: Routledge.

Salazar, M. R., T. K. Lant, S. M. Fiore, and E. Salas. 2012. "Facilitating Innovation in Diverse Science Teams through Integrative Capacity." *Small Group Research* 43: 527–58. doi: 10.1177/1046496412453622.

Tebes, J. K., and N. D. Thai. 2018. "Interdisciplinary Team Science and the Public: Steps toward a Participation Team Science." *American Psychologist* 73 (4): 549–62.

Chapter 5

Improving Racial Equity in Birth Outcomes

A Community-Based, Culturally Centered Approach

Katy Kozhimannil
University of Minnesota School of Public Health

Rachel Hardeman
University of Minnesota School of Public Health

Rebecca Polston
Roots Community Birth Center

Acknowledgment: We gratefully acknowledge the input and writing support from J'Mag Karbeah, MPH, Doctoral Student, University of Minnesota School of Public Health.

Chapter Context

Our team's goal is for African American mothers in Minneapolis and beyond to have access to care options that support a good birth. Our collective expertise includes the fields of health services research, sociology of health and illness, and critical race theory (Rachel Hardeman); midwifery, culturally centered healthcare, community advocacy (Rebecca Polston); and health policy, public policy, and statistics (Katy Kozhimannil). There are power and privilege dynamics among us and with the various audiences we wish to collaborate with and serve. To manage these challenges while conducting this research, we are committed to following principles that promote power sharing and trust building within our partnership and in interpreting findings and disseminating results among community, academic, and policy audiences.

Our three-year, collaborative research project focuses on building the evidence base around one model of care—Roots Community Birth Center—and discerning generalizable concepts, knowledge, and wisdom that may inform broader efforts toward birth equity. In our work, we are documenting the content, experiences, and outcomes of pregnancy and childbirth care provided in the context of culturally centered care. This project first described the process of care at Roots, using interviews with staff and stakeholders as well as focus group discussions with clients. We also conducted a web-based survey of all Roots clients during the postpartum period, in order to compare outcomes for Roots clients with outcomes for similar women with hospital-based care. The survey includes information on experiences of discrimination, communication, and early infant bonding in order to understand how care differs for Roots clients, compared with care that diverse patients typically receive in US hospitals. Finally it is an explicit goal of our work to communicate findings and implications broadly among those who can use this information to make personal and policy decisions to improve equity in birth outcomes.

Through this project, we have learned the potential impact of speaking truth to power and accomplishing change by targeting the clinical community through high-profile published commentaries, the payer community (through a blog series with the American Journal of Managed Care, *and in Roots' contract negotiations with health insurers), and the policy community (through engaging the media and legislation on maternal health and racism). A major lesson learned was the value of engaging on multiple fronts to achieve change. We believe that the legacy of our project is "centering at the margins" in our individual work, our collective work, and in the systems with which we engage. Centering at the margins requires reanchoring a vision of change in the lived experiences of those who have been marginalized. It necessitates redefining "normal," and it starts with ourselves and carries through all of our work.*

Introduction

People of color, African Americans in particular, have systematically worse healthcare access and outcomes, in general, and around the time of childbirth (Bryant et al. 2010; Eichelberger et al. 2016; Hogan et al. 2012). Perceived discrimination and experiences of interpersonal racism, such as selective avoidance and microaggressions, contribute to the disproportionate barriers to high-quality, respectful, patient-centered care experienced by African Americans and other people of color (Eichelberger et al. 2016; Hardeman et al. 2018; Prather et al. 2016). Current disparities are rooted in a historical context. Centuries of policies—from slavery to segregation to unethical research practices—have resulted in African American women experiencing bias and discrimination through contact with the healthcare delivery system during pregnancy and childbirth (Bridges 2011; Oparah and Bonaparte 2015). Additionally, recent research suggests that structural racism—that is, the structures, policies, practices, and norms resulting in differential access to the goods, services, and opportunities of society by race—has an impact on birth outcomes. One recent study found that there is a joint effect of income inequality and structural racism on the risk of small-for-gestational-age birth (Wallace et al. 2015).

At the same time that African Americans have suffered health burdens resulting from racism, there is also a long history of resilience. For as long as African Americans have lived in the United States, there has been a practice of culturally centered pregnancy and childbirth care, whereby African American midwives (sometimes called "granny midwives") cared for African American women outside of the medical care system. This separate care model developed out of both the strength of cultural practices and the necessity that arose from being excluded from traditional healthcare delivery systems. The medicalization of childbirth has affected African Americans and the general US population, moving 98 percent of births into hospitals; over 90 percent of births are now attended by physicians (Declercq 2015; MacDorman, Declercq, and Mathews 2013). While rates of midwife-attended births and out-of-hospital births are climbing again, the women that access these options tend to be white and upper-middle class (Declercq 2015; MacDorman et al. 2013).

One of the reasons that the rise in midwifery access is concentrated among white women is a lack of racial and ethnic diversity among midwives and few out-of-hospital birth options for African American women seeking a provider who shares their race or background (Bryant et al. 2010; Declercq 2015; Listening to Mothers III; MacDorman et al. 2013). Indeed, in their recent commentary in the *Journal of Midwifery & Women's Health*, Jennifer Foster and Jodi Delibertis stated, "The demographic profile of certified nurse-midwives, certified midwives and certified professional midwives in the United States continues to be disproportionately White" (Foster and Delibertis 2016). The prevalence of whiteness among maternity care clinicians likely pervades not just the workforce but also the culture of clinics and hospitals, where the vast majority of pregnant women receive their care. One option for out-of-hospital birth is a freestanding birth center, which is a home-like facility existing within a healthcare system with a program of care designed in the wellness model of pregnancy and birth. Pregnancy and childbirth care provided to low-risk women in freestanding birth centers compares favorably with hospital-based care and comprises a promising strategy for improving value, but little has been documented about the potential role for out-of-hospital birth to improve cultural respect and reduce disparities in childbirth care (Alliman and Phillippi 2016). Specifically, for African Americans, who experience some of the worse outcomes and highest levels of racism, access to out-of-hospital (deinstitutionalized) care from a provider that shares their cultural background may hold promise for improving both the quality and outcomes of the childbirth experience. Our collective work investigates this potential.

In Minnesota a 2015 report from the Minnesota Department of Health revealed that African American and American Indian infants are twice as likely to die in the first year of life as white infants (Minnesota Department of Health 2015). As professionals and as mothers from these communities, we know these infants and their families, and we share a commitment to narrowing this racial gap. We are engaged in dismantling racism, a critical social determinant of health, influencing inequitable childbirth outcomes (Eichelberger et al. 2016; Hardeman, Medina, and Kozhimannil 2016).

This chapter outlines our vision for a collaborative research project, which is a vehicle for achieving our shared goal of greater equity in healthy childbirth outcomes. It describes successes and challenges we have experienced within our interdisciplinary, community-based research partnership. Together, combining community knowledge, culturally-grounded competencies, and rigorous research, we believe it is possible to address the complex structural dynamics that have produced long-standing racial disparities in maternal and infant health.

Our team and research project is funded through the Robert Wood Johnson Foundation's Interdisciplinary Research Leaders (IRL) program. This three-year program funds three-person teams made up of one community partner and two academic partners, with a focus on conducting community-engaged research to advance the evidence base for creating a culture of health. The program provides funding for the research project and separate funding for a portion of time for each of us to devote to personal and professional development to improve our capacity for research leadership.

Overview of Goals

The long-term and overarching goal of this project is to produce knowledge that will help achieve racial equity in childbirth care and outcomes.
In 2014 the Minnesota Department of Health (MDH) identified structural racism as a major cause of this inequity and numerous other inequities in Minnesota (MDH 2014). Broader awareness of the link between
structural racism and health is growing, from the MDH report to the
Black Lives Matter movement. The time to participate in the creation
and dissemination of effective community-based knowledge to inform
decision-makers who care as much as we do about the children from our
communities of color having the same opportunity for a healthy start to
life as white children is now. For policymakers and others who wish to
act to improve equity, what is often lacking is a solid evidence base from
which to build successful efforts to dismantle structural racism in childbirth care and beyond.

While our project team members come from different backgrounds
and disciplines, our approach to disrupting the structural racism that
shapes early childhood begins at the same place: pregnancy. Prenatal care
is an important determinant of maternal-infant outcomes. For African
American women, however, care in the medical context is insufficient to
meet their needs. Prenatal care alone is woefully inadequate for addressing the role that structural and interpersonal racism may play in their
day-to-day experiences and their encounters with the healthcare system
(Eichelberger et al. 2016). African American women have greater barriers to access care and fewer choices for maternity care that meets their
needs (Howell et al. 2018), compared with white women.

Our work seeks to understand and articulate those needs, and to
influence the policies and structures that shape access to care to ensure

these needs are valued, honored, and met during pregnancy, childbirth, and beyond.

Theoretical Model: Racism, Weathering, and Birth Equity

Long-standing and complex sociodemographic and historical factors perpetuate the challenges African American women and other women of color face in achieving positive birth outcomes (Giscombe and Lobel 2005; Hogan 2011). Approaches aimed at achieving birth equity require an understanding of the social determinants of health—conditions in which people learn, live, work, and play (Braveman, Egerter, and Williams 2011)—and a commitment to disrupting the pathways that allow these social determinants to predispose women to adverse birth outcomes.

The weathering framework, proposed by the social scientist Arline Geronimus (1992), provides a model that explains the biological pathway through which social determinants predispose women to adverse birth outcomes. This framework tells us that health inequities between races result from exposure to social, economic, and political marginalization experienced by African Americans (compared to white Americans). This marginalization—the exclusion from mainstream social, economic, and political systems—takes many forms, including the residential segregation of African Americans into poorer quality neighborhoods, with lower access to resources such as quality schools and employment. The physical and mental health toll of this marginalization accumulates with age (Geronimus 1992; Geronimus et al. 2006) and causes biological wear and tear that makes individuals more susceptible to adverse health outcomes. Most research, intervention, and policies to address inequity in birth outcomes have focused on health behaviors and access to healthcare. A growing body of research, however, supports the argument that these "proximate" risk factors do not adequately address the dynamic and complex nature of health inequity. An alternate hypothesis, such as Geronimus's weathering framework, suggests that social context (social determinants) directly affects health. This claim is supported by a large body of literature that has documented the robust association between social determinants, such as neighborhood or socioeconomic status and health. Researchers have also documented the disparities between African Americans and whites in both the level and quality of many of these factors, including healthcare, education, income, occupation, housing, and neighborhood.

The weathering framework extends the concept of context further by asserting that health disparities can be specifically attributed to the social, economic, and political marginalization of African Americans. The extent of the health disparities reflects the level of marginalization experienced. A second component of the weathering framework suggests that the health effects of the contextual factors accumulate with age. In other words, health disparities are smaller at younger compared to older ages, reflecting the shorter cumulative exposure to these social determinants and continued exposure to various forms of marginalization.

The weathering hypothesis was empirically tested in 1996 using population-based data. Geronimus's results show that the low and very low birth weight rates for singleton first births to African American women increase with age; however, that is not the case for white women. Notably, after controlling for numerous risk factors—such as inadequate prenatal care, smoking, diabetes, hypertension, and other high-risk factors— African American women in their mid-to late twenties (conventionally considered the ideal childbearing period), still showed greater odds of low birth weight and very low birth weight compared to black women in their late teens. In other words, the black women in this study seemed to be aging at a faster rate—or weathering—than their white counterparts, as reflected in birth outcomes (Geronimus 1996).

The causes of the accelerated aging or weathering are understood to be fundamental causes—as opposed to proximate risk factors—for health inequities. The data points to racism as a fundamental cause of health inequities seen in black-white infant birth weight. Racism—a fundamental cause of health inequity—operates to make the social determinants relevant and is a key component in weathering. Although many interventions have been developed aimed at eliminating racial inequities in infant outcomes, many focus exclusively on the proximate factors and neglect racism as a fundamental cause. Unfortunately until research and interventions explicitly focus on the fundamental cause of these risk factors (racism) and attempt to eliminate its influence, new risk factors will continue to emerge to reinforce and perpetuate health inequities.

Disrupting this pathway and intervening on the fundamental cause of health inequities is a challenge that requires multi-factorial and multi-sectoral approaches. Interventions aimed at addressing racism as the fundamental cause must focus both on the interpersonal relationships African American women have with their providers but also push for structural reform that centers the needs and experiences of all marginalized populations. One model that attempts to center both interpersonal and institutional reform is that of a culturally centered freestanding birth center. This model is one element that we can explore as part of the complex effort to disrupt the pathway between racism, social determinants of health, and birth outcomes.

The Research Project

Our three-year, collaborative research project focuses on building the evidence base around one model of care—Roots Community Birth Center—and discerning generalizable concepts, knowledge, and wisdom that may inform broader efforts toward birth equity. Research in fields outside of maternity care has identified access to culturally focused care as a predictor of improved health outcomes. In our work, we are documenting the content, experiences, and outcomes of pregnancy and childbirth care provided in the context of culturally centered care. The goal of this chapter is to describe our process, including successes and challenges, in undertaking a collective, community-based research project.

This project describes the process of care at Roots Community Birth Center, using interviews with staff and stakeholders as well as focus group discussions with clients. Through analyzing data collected during interviews and focus groups, we are documenting the processes and practices for providing culturally centered care, including the distillation of key concepts and mechanisms of service delivery so that they may be more broadly replicable.

We are also conducting a web-based survey of all Roots clients during the postpartum period, in order to compare outcomes for Roots clients with outcomes for similar women with hospital-based care. The survey and comparison includes experiences of discrimination, communication, and early infant bonding in order to understand how care differs for Roots clients, compared with the care that diverse patients typically receive in US hospitals.

Finally, it is an explicit goal of our work to communicate findings and implications broadly among those who can use this information to make personal and policy decisions to improve equity in birth outcomes.

Specifically, we aim to disseminate findings to community, academic, and policy audiences, which includes pregnant residents of north Minneapolis and surrounding neighborhoods, clinicians caring for diverse pregnant patients, researchers studying birth equity, employers making decisions regarding health insurance benefits, health plan administrators making financing and coverage decisions, state and federal Medicaid program administrators, and state and federal legislators. Communicating our findings to ensure change is an essential component of our work.

Our Research Site

Roots Community Birth Center opened in 2015 in north Minneapolis, the neighborhood with the highest infant mortality rate in Minnesota. Founded by Rebecca Polston, Roots is Minnesota's first and only African American–owned and operated birth center. In establishing Roots, Polston believed she could create change in her community by creating relationships, offering employment, and training more midwives and doulas of color. This for-profit birth center is an intentional effort to bring equity and not charity to the population it serves.

The plan to develop and launch Roots was financially supported through a partnership between four community organizations: WomenVenture, Neighborhood Development Center, Northside Economic Opportunity Network, and the Minnesota Black Chamber of Commerce. With this funding, Polston established her business and hired six staff members from within the north Minneapolis community. Roots seeks to improve maternal and infant outcomes in the African American community by addressing the root—structural racism—and its corollary impact: chronic physical, psychological, and environmental stress (Geronimus et al. 2010). To do so, Roots provides culturally centered, relationship-based care to meet its clients' clinical, emotional, psychosocial, and relational needs. The hypothesized means through which the care at Roots would disrupt the manifold, pernicious consequences of racism is by centering the birthing person and harnessing the strength of their culture through the process of pregnancy and childbirth. The three of us share a commitment to the vision on which Roots was founded and have committed to a research project to document and understand its actualization, challenges, and potential. Systematically disrupting the pathways between racism and poor birth outcomes will take more than one birth center can offer, but we hope to uncover knowledge from Roots' model and approach in this research project, and to offer community wisdom into the academic and policy context of evidence for change.

Our Team

As a team, the three of us have a diverse set of talents and perspectives to support this work. Each member brings an essential skill set and perspective to achieve the goals of our proposed research project. Rachel Hardeman and Katy Kozhimannil have collaborated for seven years on both academic and community-based research projects. Our partnership was seeded four years ago when Rebecca Polston provided initial input and feedback from a cultural perspective on Kozhimannil and Hardeman's community-based doula project (Hardeman and Kozhimannil 2016; Kozhimannil et al. 2016). Over the three years, Hardeman and Polston have both been part of the establishment of the Minnesota Birth Workers of Color organization. What brought us together is a shared commitment to understanding ways to achieve equity in birth outcomes through an innovative community-based approach.

We meet in person on a monthly basis, either on campus or at Roots, and more frequently as needed. In order to balance the many competing demands on our time, but also to maintain the strength of our partnership and personal relationships, we prioritize regular, respectful, timely communication with one another via phone, text, and email, in addition to in-person meetings. Each of us takes leadership on distinct aspects of the partnership, and we return regularly to our focus and shared commitment. Later we describe both successes and challenges within our partnership, but our orienting mechanism has been shared vision, mutual respect, and specialization. That is, we continually affirm—individually and collectively—our dedication to realizing equity in childbirth, and we recognize the different strengths that each brings to the partnership.

Early Outputs, Dissemination, and Outcomes

Our overall goals are ambitious and may take longer to achieve than the three-year time frame of our current collaboration, yet we celebrate each new piece of knowledge and each product as a step along the path toward loosening the powerful grip of racism on birth outcomes. The goal of our research-dissemination plan is to raise awareness among key stakeholders about initial findings and how they may help guide the actions of policymakers to improve equity in childbirth care and outcomes in Minnesota and across the United States. As we conduct the research itself, we are focused on building strong networks for dissemination by communicating about the racial equity issues that drove us to conduct this research and relying on the expertise that each of us brings to the collaboration. We do this through our work with the media, policymakers, health plan administrators, academics, and community roles.

To date, we have created products in three major categories: community-oriented, policy-oriented, and academically oriented. Our community-oriented products and dissemination have focused on media outreach and contributing to media stories, locally and nationally, which draw attention to racial disparities in maternal and infant health, illuminate the lived experiences of people of color, and present positive alternatives and solutions to entrenched disparities.

The policy-oriented awareness work we have initiated focuses on the establishment of a blog series on the website of the *American Journal of Managed Care*, a top journal in the field of health insurance and managed care (a key audience for shifting childbirth payment policies). A blog may seem an unlikely platform for policy dissemination, but health insurance plans—including private and Medicaid–managed care organizations—are key players in maternity care payment policy. This blog series has reached our key audience for three main reasons: (1) it distills complex concepts underlying and motivating our research into accessible language and a context that is relevant for health plans, (2) it is freely publicly available and is not behind a paywall (as many academic publications are), and (3) it builds on the credibility and reach of the *American Journal of Managed Care*.

Academic publications include a case study describing the model of care provided at Roots as well as qualitative and quantitative analyses of themes that arose from survey data, focus groups, and interviews with Roots clients, staff, and stakeholders. Preliminary themes describe care that is respectful and culturally centered, and acknowledges and embraces the knowledge and lived experience of each client while also naming and actively fighting against the structural barriers within their lives by providing them with a safe space and the necessary resources.

These themes show the importance of culturally concordant care, but, more broadly, the data indicates that nonconcordant providers can provide culturally centered care when they acknowledge racism as cause of inequity and understand that reducing these inequities requires a commitment to racial justice—a commitment that often means creating space and opportunities for a more diverse maternal care workforce.

Successes

It is impossible to find words to state the depth and urgency of the personal devotion that each of us has to birth equity, and never before have we had an opportunity to work collaboratively to make a change. Our successes thus far are built on our shared commitment to this vision, and our personal commitments to one another and the people and families in our communities whose lives have been unmistakably altered by experiences of structural and interpersonal racism during pregnancy and birth.

Interestingly, our successes in this project have not taken the typical form expected of and anticipated from large, national grants. Rather than having a long list of academic manuscripts, our successes have taken the form of visibility and dialogue in the media, giving voice to women's stories, engagement in policy discussions, mentorship, and personal growth.

To that end, as we collaborate on our research project, we look ahead to the transformation toward greater access to culturally centered care as we: (1) uncover the tenets of this care concept, (2) work to support maternity care payment reform that rewards quality over quantity, and (3) support the recruitment and retention of a diverse maternity care workforce. Additionally, we continue to draw attention to the foundational need to address structural racism as an underlying cause of birth inequities.

Visibility and Dialogue in the Media

The core work of this project is not just the process of collecting and analyzing data but in communicating findings and implications broadly among those who can use it to make personal and policy decisions to improve equity in birth outcomes. One of the most meaningful successes of our collective work has been the opportunity to engage with media— locally, statewide, and nationally—to share our vision and to connect our goals with the lived experiences of women and families of color. For example, in the summer of 2017 the Minnesota *Spokesman-Recorder* did an in-depth, two-part story about Roots Community Birth Center, the need for more midwives of color, the goals of our research, and the urgent challenge of racial disparities in birth care and outcomes in north Minneapolis. The Minnesota *Spokesman-Recorder*, established in 1934, is the oldest African American–owned newspaper in the state of Minnesota and one of the longest-standing, family-owned newspapers in the United States. As such, having our work highlighted by this publication was deeply meaningful to engaging directly in the community where we hope to have the greatest impact.

At the national level, Hardeman and Kozhimannil have had the opportunity to contribute to the background and to share our own research to shape media coverage of the racial equity aspects of the maternal mortality crisis. Speaking directly with reporters and providing them with detailed information has an impact on how women's stories are told and woven together. It is deeply important to us that, given the pervasiveness of racism, the tender and vulnerable stories of maternal and infant loss in the African American community are not tokenized or stylized, but that they reflect the richness of the lived experiences and honor the tragedies that people have endured.

Additionally, our team has worked with a photojournalist to share the story of Roots. In April 2018 Black Maternal Health Week was a national effort to draw attention to the disproportionate vulnerability that African American women, infants, and families experience around the time of pregnancy and childbirth. Through our work with media, we were able to help amplify attention to these issues on social media and also to shape the stories being told by sharing our data and connecting journalists with women who have stories to share. For example, both Kozhimannil and Hardeman spoke with Nina Martin, a journalist at ProPublica, who won a Peabody Award for her co-leadership of a project on maternal mortality called "Lost Mothers." In our conversations with Martin, we were able to emphasize the links between structural racism and maternal mortality and encourage her to address these directly. Indeed, she did exactly this in a December 2017 article titled, "Nothing Protects Black Women from Dying in Pregnancy and Childbirth," highlighting the story of Shalon Irving, who died early in 2017, shortly after giving birth to her daughter, Soleil. Since Martin and her colleagues published this piece, both Hardeman and Kozhimannil continue to be in touch with her and with other journalists who are interested in highlighting stories of inequity in birth.

Giving Voice to Women's Stories

Our initial data collection and findings from focus group discussions and interviews have created an archive of important and impactful narratives of the lived experiences of African American women—and their families—who are participating in culturally centered care during pregnancy and birth. When describing her birth experience, one participant remarked:

> I felt like it was too much because I didn't know what pushing felt like. Rebecca said, "Take your time, I'm not rushing you... Ok, you're pushing!" After that, [my baby's] head came out and it was the strongest contraction I ever had in my life. I looked at Rebecca and she said, "Now catch her." I said, "I'm not catching her, I can't do this." It's what I said... you know, send me to the hospital... just send me to the hospital. And she just looked at me so calmly, like just caring. Like a mother, a natural feeling. And she just said, "Just push. Like you have to yell." I yelled and the baby came out on the second push. I'm proud of having the baby, honestly.

This quote was one of many that highlight the immense support women note having at Roots as well as the control they feel during their laboring process. We see a paradigm shift in this participant's ability to see her child's birth as something she accomplished rather than a task accomplished by her provider. These are the narratives that have the power to shift the culture of health when effectively communicated to a range of stakeholders—from policymakers to clinicians to healthcare delivery systems administrators to employers to health plans. Our work with the media is one way in which we have had success, but the research itself—from interviews to surveys to focus group discussions—is elevating stories of extraordinary empowerment. Bearing witness to and recording these transcendent moments of physical and emotional transformation is a deep honor. So often the media portrayals of African American childbirth show the tragic side of how racism affects care and outcomes. In this project we hear, again and again, positive stories of African American childbirth, and we are aggregating and analyzing women's stories to understand the common threads of their experiences of culturally centered care.

Engagement in Policy Discussions

Once we are able to uncover these positive stories, it is essential to translate these not only to the general public and to the community where we work but also to policymakers and others with the power to make decisions that shape the opportunities that women have for a safe, healthy childbirth. Our partnership and project is creating a pathway for those in positions of privilege and power to learn from those with wisdom and knowledge that is critical to the success and efficacy of public policies, especially payment policies, aimed to set children and families on the right track from the moment of birth, and over the life course. For example, as mentioned earlier, to inform health plans and managed-care organizations about aspects of maternity care reimbursement that could contribute to greater equity, we established a blog series on the *American Journal of Managed Care*'s website. We have had extensive traffic to these posts, especially "How Health Plans Can Support Moms" and "As We Mourn Infant Death, Let's Take Care of Moms," along with "Our Maternity Care System Is Broken: Here's How We Can Fix It." Polston recently successfully used the blog posts to support her discussions regarding reimbursement with a local health plan. Additionally, both Hardeman and Kozhimannil have provided input to federal legislators on proposed policies that relate to maternal mortality, and Kozhimannil provided testimony on a bill in the Minnesota legislature that would designate funding within the state's broader equity initiatives to focus on racial disparities in prenatal care. In December 2018 the Preventing Maternal Deaths Act, a federal bill designed to support a maternal mortality review infrastructure in every state, was signed into law. Importantly this legislation encourages representation of communities most affected by maternal mortality, including black women.

Mentorship

In addition to successes in outward impacts, we have reflected on feelings of success that relate to interpersonal relationships as well as building the future workforce in our fields. Mentorship has a critical role in the way that our research team operates and is successful. Relying loosely on a cascade framework in which knowledge and experience flow from the most senior to the most junior, our team is composed not just of the two researchers and community partner—we also include a high school student, a midwifery student, and a doctoral student. All three student partners are involved in every aspect of the project and have taken the lead on coding a majority of the qualitative data.

Through our project, our high school student has developed leadership skills that have translated into discussing issues of race and gender among her classmates and school leadership. She has presented her work on this project at her school's science fair and as a culminating experience for her advanced science research course. She has grown as a leader and has strengthened her ability to critically analyze issues; also, her work has been instrumental in our project. She began her freshman year at Yale University in the fall of 2018. She begins her undergraduate career having been trained in quantitative and qualitative methodology but, most importantly, is intimately familiar with the ability of community-led, woman-led, and people-of-color-led organizations to uplift and eliminate inequities within their own communities.

Our midwifery student recently graduated, becoming one of only seven midwives of color in Minnesota. She recently joined the academic faculty at the University of Minnesota, where she practices midwifery and conducts research related to reproductive health outcomes. She was recruited for the position in part due to her role as a researcher on our project. Our doctoral student has taken the lead on conducting and leading focus groups and writing manuscripts. As a scholar of color in the field of health services research, we are intentionally preparing her for a successful career in academia. Additionally, her experience working alongside a community partner has given her the research experience that is not only professionally desirable but will allow her to advocate for similar projects in her training and career.

Personal Growth

We are grateful for the tremendous personal growth that has accompanied our work on this project and on these issues. This work has not been easy (more on that shortly), but facing these challenges individually and as a team has influenced each of us.

We gratefully recognize the position of privilege and power we hold as recipients of a major national grant, and by virtue of our positions as professionals. This recognition is a gift, as it allows us to harness our own agency in the face of the impacts of persistent racism in our communities and in our own lives. The close proximity to those who have experienced maternal or infant mortality and those who are struggling to care for themselves and their families during pregnancy and childbirth have clarified for us the value of the credentials we have earned, elevating the urgency of our work to address racial disparities in childbirth.

This research collaboration and partnership have added credibility to our voices that we can use in new and unique ways to influence knowledge (especially Hardeman), policy (especially Kozhimannil), and clinical practice (especially Polston). Additionally, through a success that we have achieved, finding a way to specialize as teammates and to work with others who respectfully challenge us, we have each developed some humility about the limits of our knowledge and understanding. Finally, we are grateful for the camaraderie we have built in facing the depth of challenge presented by antiracism work, including mutual respect for the need for self-care.

Challenges

Our different perspectives are our strength, but they also present challenges. We have trained in different fields. We bring different personal and professional experiences and expectations and—importantly—we face different constraints and incentives in our professional environments. In our collaborative work, we have faced challenges in setting expectations, time management, meeting externally imposed criteria for success, and financial sustainability.

Setting Expectations and Time Management

We come to this project with different backgrounds and different exposure to the professions of academia and small business ownership and to the fields of research and midwifery. Coming together from a university and community perspective was—and continues to be—a challenge for us. Both setting and articulating expectations required more time and attention than we anticipated, and each of us had unarticulated assumptions that needed to be challenged.

The challenge of setting expectations and the time required for relationship-building, trust, and deliberative discussion, which are required for collaborative decision-making and co-ownership of the work, was exacerbated for us by the many competing priorities that we each have in our personal and professional lives. For example, the pace and requirements of research differ immensely from the pace and tenor of midwifery work, which—by its very nature—is unpredictable and high intensity. Balancing our individual workloads in a way that supports our collective work has been a challenge.

Meeting Externally Imposed Criteria for Success

Additionally, each of us—in our professional roles—has externally imposed criteria for success, and these criteria differ among us. Specifically, Polston is the owner of a for-profit business and, as a businesswoman, needs to attend to the needs of her clients, staff, and operations. Also, Hardeman is a tenure-track faculty member whose progress toward tenure is annually assessed—her contract renewal is dependent on how tenured faculty assess and vote on the value of her work over the prior year. Kozhimannil is a tenured faculty member but also remains in a soft-money academic environment, where the imperative to generate salary support through grant funding and to publish prolifically in peer-reviewed journals remains paramount. The transformative work that this project requires is frequently not directly contributing to many of the expectations we need to meet in order to advance or sustain our professional work.

This has manifested in dropping planned products, either because they do not meet the immediate needs of our community or because they do not meet the expectations required for professional advancement on the tenure track or the business needs of a birth center. Our ability to manage these challenges has depended on the strength of our personal relationships and honest discussions with one another—including a willingness to be vulnerable to share and to listen.

Financial Sustainability of the Birth Center Model of Care

With a commitment to providing relationship-based, culturally centered care, open to all potential clients, Roots has faced serious financial challenges to support its model of care. This is directly relevant to one shared goal of our work: ensuring financial sustainability for a model of care that honors culture and overcomes racial disparities.

For example, clinic-based maternity care is reimbursed as a single payment for all prenatal and postpartum visits. Extra time spent is not reimbursed, but extra procedures, tests, and laboratory results are. In the Roots model, it is not uncommon to provide thirteen to fifteen prenatal visits, each lasting thirty to ninety minutes. Visits go beyond the usual tests and include time-intensive services, such as nutritional counseling, care coordination, and family support. In the current maternity care financing model, the Roots model is not well supported, adding strain on staff and resources, which limits Rebecca's time for research collaboration, and calls into question the premise of whether the level of transformation we envision is possible. We are working to change policies, but change is not coming fast enough for Roots.

Principles for Building on Success to Meet the Challenges We Face

In our collaborative work, we aim to manage our challenges by abiding by the following guidelines in maintaining trust and partnership among members of our team: (1) starting conversations about our partnership early, (2) clearly identifying priorities of each partner, (3) clearly identifying the goals of the project, (4) openly discussing prior experiences—positive or negative—with collaborative and research partnerships, and (5) assuming good intentions and making good on our commitments. Further, there are power and privilege dynamics among us and with the various audiences we wish to reach with our work. To manage the challenges that relate to power and privilege in the conduct of this research, we are committed to the following principles to promote power sharing within our partnership, and as we interpret findings and disseminate results among community, academic, and policy audiences: (1) reflect on and acknowledge socially defined power differentials, (2) strive to lessen impact of privilege by creating an equitable partnership, (3) acknowledge and value the expertise and skills of all partners, (4) emphasize needs identified by community, and (5) spend time on relationships with each other and with the target audiences of our work.

However, there is little we can do on a daily basis to transform the enormous obstacles on our progress that are created by historical and contemporary manifestations of structural racism in policies and institutions, including the places where we work and live. Yet we continue to strive toward greater equity, and we believe it is a goal worth fighting for.

References

Alliman, J., and J. C. Phillippi. 2016. "Maternal Outcomes in Birth Centers: An Integrative Review of the Literature." *Journal of Midwifery & Women's Health* 61 (1): 21–51.

American Association of Birth Centers. http://www.birthcenters.org.

Braveman, P., S. Egerter, and D. R. Williams. 2011. "The Social Determinants of Health: Coming of Age." *Annual Review of Public Health* 32: 381–98.

Bridges, K. 2011. *Reproducing Race: An Ethnography of Pregnancy as a Aite of Racialization*. Berkeley: University of California Press.

Bryant, A. S., A. Worjoloh, A. B. Caughey, and A. E. Washington. 2010. "Racial/ Ethnic Disparities in Obstetric Outcomes and Care: Prevalence and Determinants." *American Journal of Obstetrics and Gynecology* 202 (4): 335–43.

Declercq, E. 2015. "Midwife-Attended Births in the United States, 1990–2012: Results from Revised Birth Certificate Data." *Journal of Midwifery & Women's Health* 60 (1): 10–15.

Eichelberger, K. Y., K. Doll, G. E. Ekpo, and M. L. Zerden. 2016a. "Black Lives Matter: Claiming a Space for Evidence-Based Outrage in Obstetrics and Gynecology." *American Journal of Public Health* 106 (10): 1771–72.

Foster, J., and J. Delibertis. 2016. "Making Midwifery a Diverse and Inclusive Profession: What's Our Story?" *Journal of Midwifery & Women's Health* 61 (6): 690–93.

Geronimus, A. T. 1992. "The Weathering Hypothesis and the Health of African-American Women and Infants: Evidence and Speculations." *Ethnicity & Disease* 2 (3): 207–21.

Geronimus, A. T. 1996. "Black/White Differences in the Relationship of Maternal Age to Birthweight: A Population-Based Test of the Weathering Hypothesis." *Social Science & Medicine* 42 (4): 589–97.

Geronimus, A. T., M. T. Hicken, D. Keene, and J. Bound. 2006. "Weathering and Age Patterns of Allostatic Load Scores among Blacks and Whites in the United States." *American Journal of Public Health* 96 (5): 826–33.

Geronimus, A. T., M. T. Hicken, J. A. Pearson, S. J. Seashols, K. L. Brown, and T. D. Cruz. 2010. "Do US Black Women Experience Stress-Related Accelerated Biological Aging?" *Human Nature* 21 (1): 19–38.

Giscombe, C. L., and M. Lobel. 2005. "Explaining Disproportionately High Rates of Adverse Birth Outcomes among African Americans: The Impact of Stress, Racism, and Related Factors in Pregnancy." *Psychological Bulletin* 131 (5): 662–83.

Hardeman, R. R., and K. B. Kozhimannil. 2016. "Motivations for Entering the Doula Profession: Perspectives from Women of Color." *Journal of Midwifery & Women's Health* 61 (6): 773–80.

Hardeman, R. R., E. M. Medina, and K. B. Kozhimannil. 2016. "Structural Racism and Supporting Black Lives: The Role of Health Professionals." *New England Journal of Medicine* 375 (22): 2113–15.

Hardeman, R. R., K. A. Murphy, J. M. Karbeah, and K. B. Kozhimannil. 2018. "Naming Institutionalized Racism in the Public Health Literature: A Systematic Literature Review." *Public Health Reports* 133 (3): 240–49.

Hogan, V., D. Rowley, T. Bennett, and K. Taylor. 2012. "Life Course, Social Determinants, and Health Inequities: Toward a National Plan for Achieving Health Equity for African American Infants—A Concept Paper." *Maternal and Child Health Journal* 16 (6): 1143–50.

Hogan, V. K., M. E. Shanahan, and D. L. Rowley. 2011. "Current Approaches to Reducing Premature Births and Implications for Disparity Elimination." In *Reducing Racial/Ethnic Disparities in Reproductive and Perinatal Outcomes: The Evidence from Population-Based Interventions*, edited by A. K. Handler and J. Peacock, 181–207. New York: Springer.

Howell, E. A., H. Brown, J. Brumley, A. S. Bryant, A. B. Caughey, A. M. Cornell, J. H. Grant, K. D. Gregory, S. M. Gullo, K. B. Kozhimannil, J. M. Mhyre, P. Toledo, R. D. Oria, M. Ngoh, and W. A. Grobman. 2018. "Reduction of Peripartum Racial and Ethnic Disparities: A Conceptual Framework and Maternal Safety Consensus Bundle." *Journal of Midwifery & Women's Health* 63 (3): 366–76.

Kozhimannil, K. B., C. A. Vogelsang, R. R. Hardeman, and S. Prasad. 2016. "Disrupting the Pathways of Social Determinants of Health: Doula Support during Pregnancy and Childbirth." *Journal of the American Board of Family Medicine* 29 (3): 308–17.

Listening to Mothers III. http://transform.childbirthconnection.org/reports/listening tomothers/.

MacDorman, M. F., E. Declercq, and T. Mathews. 2013. "Recent Trends in Out-of-Hospital Births in the United States." *Journal of Midwifery & Women's Health* 58 (5): 494–501.

Minnesota Department of Health (MDH). 2014. *Advancing Health Equity in Minnesota: Report to the Legislature*. https://www.health.state.mn.us/communities/equity/reports/ahe_leg_report_020114.pdf.

Minnesota Department of Health. 2015. *Infant Mortality Reduction Plan for Minnesota*. https://www.health.state.mn.us/docs/people/womeninfants/infantmort/infant mortality.pdf.

Oparah, J. C., and A. D. Bonaparte. 2015. *Birthing Justice: Black Women, Pregnancy, and Childbirth*. New York: Routledge.

Prather, C., T. R. Fuller, K. J. Marshall, and W. L. Jeffries. 2016. "The Impact of Racism on the Sexual and Reproductive Health of African American Women." *Journal of Women's Health* 25 (7): 664–71.

Wallace, M. E., P. Mendola, D. Liu, and K. L. Grantz. 2015. "Joint Effects of Structural Racism and Income Inequality on Small-for-Gestational-Age Birth." *American Journal of Public Health* 105 (8): 1681–88.

Chapter 6

Creating Transformational Nonprofit/ University Partnerships in Public Health

Lessons Derived from Collaboration between Room to Grow and Columbia University

Allyson Crawford
Room to Grow

Bethany C. Brichta
Room to Grow

Ruby L. Engel
Center on Poverty and Social Policy, Columbia University School of Social Work

Joanna Groccia
Room to Grow

Anna E. Holt
Room to Grow

Tonya Pavlenko
Center on Poverty and Social Policy, Columbia University School of Social Work

Karen Juliet Sanchez
Center on Poverty and Social Policy, Columbia University School of Social Work

Christopher Wimer
Center on Poverty and Social Policy, Columbia University School of Social Work

Chapter Context

The research team from Columbia University and the director of Room to Grow have been in the field together on this project since 2015. Room to Grow is a nonprofit organization that offers structured coaching, material goods, and community connections to support parents in activating their natural strengths and expand their knowledge, so their children thrive from the start. Room to Grow has been partnering with families and children since 1998. Together the research team and community partner believe that effective collaboration between academia and nonprofit organizations, doing direct work in communities, is crucial to achieving broad and transformational social change.

This chapter details how the members built a successful nonprofit/university partnership to show that innovative early childhood programs that combine income supports, parenting education, and connections to community services promote early childhood health and development. The team piloted a research-informed program model that combines tailored, one-on-one in-person sessions between an expectant mother and an expert clinical social worker. In addition to the social worker sessions, which occurred every three months, expectant mothers had ongoing communication by phone and email with the Room to Grow staff, were provided essential baby items, and connected to vital community resources. The pilot was designed to be upscaled into a larger demonstration project if successful outcomes were established.

This chapter outlines the questions and challenges the team wrestled with along the way as they designed and implemented a complex research project. The team also introduces their current plan to disseminate findings from the research effort and Room to Grow's philosophy of social service delivery— the combination of social supports with material supports—that could have broad, cross-sector applications.

Introduction

One of the most challenging strategic problems for nonprofit organizations in the twenty-first century is balancing excellent direct program services that achieve social impact with research and evaluation to continuously improve these programs and effectively communicate impact to external audiences. While the use of data to drive program improvement and organizational learning should be a priority for any nonprofit, resource generation (i.e., raising money and in-kind support) is also key to achieving long-term financial sustainability. In the current philanthropic climate, data and evaluation play a major role in an organization's ability to sustain itself and truly achieve social change through innovation. In order to answer the call for rigorous evidence, organizations often need to look outside of their staff and beyond their own knowledge base and form carefully crafted research partnerships. Sophisticated partnership between nonprofits and research organizations, such as universities, is the linchpin at the center of this data challenge. Unfortunately at the heart of most university and nonprofit relationships are gaps in common experiences, tensions around time and other resources, and philosophical differences that oftentimes position direct service work in opposition to academic structure, rigor, and culture. Yet even in the face of these challenges, some partnerships rise to the top, creating unique and pivotal examples of transformational change that can emerge from a shared understanding of both academic and real-life context with a common vision for social impact. In this chapter, our aim is to convey our experience of a hard-won, long-term successful partnership between a nonprofit and a university in the hope that others may move toward similarly meaningful and effective relationships that advance the nonprofit sector in tangible ways. This narrative reflection case study has been composed by numerous members of our teams—both Room to Grow staff and Columbia University researchers—who offer insight into their experiences of the project.

Over the last several years, Room to Grow—a comprehensive, strengths-based, two-generation program for parents of children under the age of three, currently located in New York City and Boston—and Columbia University have built a partnership and cultivated a vision for shared impact. We hope that our experience in this partnership will leave a legacy of learning and development that will inform the fields of social services, early childhood education, and academia over the long haul. In that spirit, we hope that our experiences may yield useful information, both strategic and brass tacks, about how to implement partnerships that will help to move other mission-based and academic endeavors forward.

The Room to Grow Program

Our program delivers three critical supports—parent coaching, essential baby goods and gear, and service referrals—to babies and their families living in poverty. Families are referred to Room to Grow during a mother's third trimester by community members, including Room to Grow program graduates, and a network of partner hospitals, prenatal clinics, and community-based organizations working with low-income families. Potential program participants may also refer themselves directly.

One-on-one parent coaching is provided during quarterly sessions with clinical and community staff members at our family center from the mother's third trimester to the child's third birthday (thirteen visits). We are committed to offering a positive and dignified experience to all families and embrace a distinctive philosophy: a therapeutic, strengths-based approach to creating sustainable, long-term change in the lives of parents and their children. Our site-based operating model is an integral part of the clinical philosophy and critical to our program's success. Room to Grow's family center welcomes families into a nurturing, child-centered space—a safe haven from the many day-to-day challenges of living in poverty. Often trust begins to build the moment a new family walks through the door. In addition to discussions on parenting strategies and child development, clinicians also offer emotional support to families and help parents develop adaptive coping skills to effectively manage life's stressors, which are particularly acute for families living in poverty.

Room-to-Grown provides referrals to community resources in order to further facilitate stability in families. Referrals are individualized to each family's needs and tailored to help families reach their short- and long-term goals. Clinicians coach families on how to access vital resources and assist them in navigating a matrix of services such as early intervention, housing, job/education referrals, and mental health support. At every visit, parents are guided as they co-select baby goods—for example, books, toys, clothing, and equipment—that support the specific areas of learning and development discussed in the session. These materials constitute an average retail value of $10,000 over the three-year period. Between in-person visits, staff members use technology to stay in touch with families, leveraging technology to celebrate and build on progress and to address new questions and ongoing concerns. We currently have two program sites in Boston and one in New York City, reaching nearly 1,000 families in total. We have plans to grow our presence in these two cities to touch over 2,500 families in the next few years, and we have aspirations to expand even more in the future.

Building Evaluation Partnerships

Running a randomized control trial (RCT) of a nonprofit organization is a trial within itself. The level of precision within a codified curriculum, programmatic operations, and team culture that is required in order to seamlessly implement this kind of research is far more than we could have imagined in the early stages of our project. Additionally, the sensitivity of the partnership between an organization's leadership and a principal investigator (PI) is beyond what could be described in these pages. At the beginning of our partnership we thought that doing a research project would make sense primarily because we have an excellent program model but also because a study could advance the field and push forward concepts that have yet to be considered comprehensively.

We also believed it could help procure funding for this type of model and our organization long-term and at scale. Three years later—and halfway through the implementation of the RCT—we have realized that meaningful engagement with a research partner requires an investment far beyond typical professional endeavors. In the following pages we outline specific examples where the advice, support, and nonjudgmental culture—the fabric of our partnership with Columbia University—improved our curriculum, operations, and efficiency as an organization, advancing the quality of our programming. In addition to laying the groundwork for a high-quality, rigorous RCT design this process ensured that our project included a viable implementation methodology, taking into consideration the realities of running a program on the ground with a population facing numerous, complex social and financial challenges. In hindsight, this value add has become extremely apparent. Along the way there were inflection points where it seemed that this project might not go as smoothly as we had hoped. The solutions involved risk-taking, compromise, allowance for misunderstanding, and frequent communion. Our joint commitment to the well-being of families and their babies ultimately brought us together to make best-in-class, high-stakes decisions about research methodologies, standardization of practice, and exceptions to the rules that may bring research rigor into question but prioritized the moral imperative of supporting the advancement of the human condition for each study participant.

For nearly twenty years, Room to Grow has been doing good work with families from low-income communities, but the information we had been using to report success only included inputs and dosage metrics—the number of clinical hours spent with families and the material goods (e.g., number of baby books) distributed to families—rather than outputs or true impact measures, which would indicate the achievement—or lack thereof—of social change. In order for Room to Grow to develop, the staff knew they needed a formal research and evaluation plan. For the last five years, finding a pathway to rigorously evaluating impact was a fundamental priority of the organization.

Through a network of connections, the Room to Grow director (first author of this chapter) began meeting with Dr. Jane Waldfogel at Columbia's School of Social Work. After reviewing Room to Grow's model together, she immediately expressed interest in conducting research on our program and suggested that the primary means to do so was likely an RCT. Waldfogel quickly brought on her colleague, Dr. Jeanne Brooks-Gunn, a giant in the field of early learning and a faculty member at Columbia's Teachers College. They had long imagined a program model that conjoined financial supports with parenting supports under a theory that the combined value of those interventions would be worth more than the sum of their parts. Their previous research seemed to point in that direction, but they had never found an early childhood program that played to both strengths until they discovered Room to Grow (Chaudry and Wimer 2016; Yeung, Linver, and Brooks-Gunn 2002; Brooks-Gunn and Duncan 1997). Waldfogel and Brooks-Gunn helped elucidate the transformational value of combining social supports and parenting supports within the organically derived Room to Grow model. At that point Room to Grow had not worked with external partners to design research measuring the intervention's effectiveness. To consider a full-scale RCT was a stretch for the organization at that stage, both in terms of having an academic understanding of research design and having the resources it would require on-the-ground for implementation. At the same time, it was clear that there was a shared understanding of the value and innovative nature of the model and a collective interest in further pursuing a rigorous evaluation project with two leading researchers in our field—an opportunity we could not pass up.

Our exploratory RCT is designed to test the effectiveness of the combination of social supports and material support in one delivery model. Participants were randomized prior to learning whether they would be part of the treatment or control group and all potential participants were given the opportunity to opt-out of the study without impacting their chances of obtaining a slot in the program. Over a one-and-a-half-year period, Columbia researchers interviewed all treatment and control group families with in-person, in-home surveys before their children's birth. Ongoing data collection follows families annually for the first three years of their children's lives (the duration of Room to Grow program participation).

Before explaining the process of implementing our RCT and corresponding learnings, we want to address the moral challenges inherent to the application of an RCT study to a community-based program. While in hindsight there are a number of ways that we would have improved our work with the community, we strongly stand behind our decision to implement an RCT over other research design options (e.g., quasi-experimental). One primary factor in this decision is that our population of families, while they touch many other systems in some cases, fall through the cracks of national and local support systems in general (Citizens' Committee for Children 2015). There is no one place, no National Office of Families with Young Children, where low-income families with young children can access comprehensive supports from pregnancy until they enter the K–12 education system, which itself is limited. This makes it particularly hard to evaluate the success of birth-to-three interventions without an RCT and corresponding control group. The primary conundrum with a control group is that researchers are determining through a lottery system who receives services and who does not, as dictated by the research methodology. If there is a slot open in a program and a potential participant is randomized into the control group, that person misses out on what could constitute life-changing supports. In order to address this moral conundrum, we decided to launch our RCT only when program slots were filled and the organization carried a waiting list; randomization was only carried out when there was one open slot and two potential participants. At times when there were unfilled slots in the program, we paused the randomization process until participation was maxed out once again in order to ensure equity. In many cases, the control group has benefitted from interactions with our Columbia research team, including receiving small cash incentives and a basket of baby items for their participation, referrals to other resources in extreme cases, and sometimes experiencing relief from social isolation when participating in interviews. The reality of this design is that the control group is receiving some support from our team, which could arguably reduce the variation we expect to see between treatment (program participants) and control (nonprogram participants) groups, albeit to a small degree. In the early days of our partnership, academic and community partners spent many hours wrestling with these inherent tensions between service and research goals. We weighed different options for design, carefully considered what would constitute a fair and valid methodology and, in the end, stand behind our hard-won decisions about what's best for participating families in the short-term and the transformational value that could be experienced by countless families across the country over time if we're able to prove the effectiveness of and scale this innovative model. In addition to this approach to randomization, we have also added qualitative elements to our research design, converting our project to a mixed-methods approach, which we expect will yield nuanced insights into the experience of participants in the project and help us to draw more accurate and nuanced conclusions about what works.

Early on we formed a rare, but effective, tripod project team. Room to Grow brought programmatic and clinical expertise as well as our unique program model with its research-informed curriculum. Waldfogel and the Columbia School of Social Work contributed their deep knowledge about poverty and the impact of public policies on child and family well-being. Finally Brooks-Gunn and the Columbia Teachers College brought their expertise in early childhood development, particularly the way in which family conditions influence how young children thrive. We received a grant from the Robert Wood Johnson Foundation (RWJF), an institution with a vision to build a culture of health, which was a perfect match for our project, as it related to the social determinants of population-level health outcomes. To begin the project Waldfogel brought in her right-hand man, Dr. Christopher Wimer, a senior research scientist and co-director of the Center on Poverty and Social Policy at the Columbia University School of Social Work. Years later, through our partnership and joint fellowship with the RWJF, the team is proud to call Wimer a friend and a partner. Together we have devised a rigorous and practical research project that has helped to hone the Room to Grow program model and has clarified our philosophy of social change. We continue to weather the challenges of implementing a rigorous research project, raising money for it, and managing budgets that demanded tough choices. In the following pages, we outline examples of the aforementioned themes and important lessons learned that advanced both our programmatic work and our research. We look forward to the continued evolution of our partnership and developing new insights over the years to come.

Lessons Learned through Study Design and Process Evaluation

The design and planning period leading up to the start of study enroll-ment challenged the Room to Grow team to carefully review all the internal program operations, policies, and unwritten norms that had existed for years, with an eye for clarity, efficiency, and standardization. This review process—which preceded the RWJF funding—not only prepared Room to Grow for a smooth rollout of the RCT and increased our capabilities to provide process evaluation data but also set us up to more effectively onboard new clinical staff, open new program sites, and replicate the program with fidelity to the model.

The core of Room to Grow's programming is the individualized parent coaching that families receive at each visit. The goal has always been to meet families where they are and to tailor visits to their needs (Flacks and Boynton-Jarrett 2018; Wilson-Simmons, Jiang, and Aratani 2017). Clinicians facilitate sessions guided by the program's curriculum, which is written to enable them to use their discretion and focus their coaching on the supports that families need the most. Visit data was his-torically collected and recorded on paper forms, making it onerous—and sometimes nearly impossible—to lift key data points for reporting dosage fidelity and outcomes in a standardized way. Using the program curric-ulum as a starting point, the Room to Grow team embarked on a transi-tion away from paper forms toward standardized, easily reportable data collection by identifying key metrics to be tracked during each program visit—ranging from demographic information such as living situation or change in employment status, to assessing whether a child's development was on track. Once these metrics were identified, we set out to program the data capture into a simple, electronic format. Room to Grow already used case management software to house basic information about families

enrolled in the program (e.g., contact information, demographics, scheduled appointments, visits notes). One of the most challenging components
of our planning for evaluation was to ensure that Room to Grow was
committed to standardized internal data collection while, at the same
time, making it as manageable as possible for the staff to record the data.
With the help of an external consultant, we were able to build out our
existing infrastructure to mirror the format of each visit's curriculum and
then create user-friendly electronic forms where clinicians could capture
their notes and data in real time. Practitioners were consulted throughout
the conversion process and played a crucial role in piloting and improving the technology to match their practice. A critical investment in tablet
technology and a handheld stylus allowed clinicians to seamlessly fill out
these forms during the visit, maintaining the comfortable feel of hand-
written note-taking and allowing them to move around a room with a
family and child. Once electronic forms are submitted, all recorded data
automatically maps to the corresponding meeting record in the database,
which eliminates the need for any manual entry. Clinicians are asked to
review their data daily and weekly through an automatically generated
report showing any holes in the information they've submitted during
their sessions, ensuring ongoing data integrity.

In addition to the standardization of curriculum data points using
electronic capture, we also built out custom technology to track program
dosage that occurs in between formal program visits. Families often
keep in close contact with their clinician if they have questions or need
additional support. Knowing that this dosage data would be important
for process evaluation, we built out additional custom infrastructure
for collecting, categorizing, and logging all contact that clinicians have
with families. Similarly, the family's electronic record includes a designated place for logging any referrals that the Room to Grow staff make

to external supports—early intervention, mental health services, legal support, etc.—as well as short- and long-term goals that families set throughout their time in the program. Clinicians are easily able to check in on these referrals and goals and provide any additional support that a family may need throughout the three years of the program. Anecdotally, we knew that these referrals and goal-setting conversations were happening with families, but planning for evaluation charged us to create solutions for formally tracking these key components of our model.

While the transition to electronic capture required quite a bit of planning and training, it ultimately improved our ability to report on program quality and outcomes even in the short term and gave us access to new data that helps us better understand our participants and their needs. We can also now access this information with the click of a button—something that previously required days of manual coding. With all this new data at our fingertips also came the challenge of monitoring what was being collected for both quality and completion. Our questions around what our internal data monitoring system should look like arose around the same time that we began discussing RCT process evaluation. In order to track the program dosage for families in the treatment group, our two teams worked together to develop a comprehensive process evaluation report. This report looks at key, internally collected Room to Grow data that provides insight into program fidelity and dosage across study participants. To build the report, we sat down with Columbia to review the data points already required at each visit and discuss whether or not additional information would be necessary when conducting formal research. The Columbia team offered helpful suggestions, such as adding an open text box for clinicians to provide context when the recommended content in the curriculum was not covered in the course of a visit. This provides additional insight during internal data review and is also in alignment with our philosophy of giving clinicians discretion over covering the curriculum in response to each family's individual needs.

Once all of the fields were agreed on and established, we then programmed a report in Room to Grow's family database that pulled all relevant fields from treatment case visits for a certain period of time. This made it easy to format and pass along process data to the team at Columbia for their own use, but it also was a natural starting point to enhance our own internal data monitoring. We began using this same report to ensure that each clinician was maintaining complete and clean data by auto generating weekly reports that prompt them to review their visits from the previous week and fill any gaps that they may have missed during sessions to achieve compliance. Columbia's advice and ideas based on their experience with process evaluation proved invaluable as we developed our own organization-wide program-monitoring systems, especially as we achieved a large enough volume of consistent data to review and analyze for quality-improvement purposes.

Learning and implementing new technology also generated ideas about how to better manage data from our external partners. Prior to the RCT, Room to Grow solicited and processed program referrals much like other small, social service organizations: by taking referrals over the phone or via fax. This practice was time- and labor-intensive for our clinical team as well as for those sending in referrals. Working through a stack of paper intake forms also meant that referrals were often processed on a delay. Additionally, the manual process inadvertently created inequity within our program intake process since clinicians were free to make subjective judgments on eligibility. It also did not help in debunking the "creaming myth" that often came up in conversations with funders and donors—the idea that we were selecting families who were more likely to be successful in our program, or perhaps those who were less in need of services, rather than first-come, first-served enrollment. We needed to standardize our process, especially since variability would be unacceptable during a rigorous research trial.

Once again we began by incorporating a technology-based solution to reduce the need for manual administrative work. Using the same form technology as the curriculum data capture, we created an electronic version of our referral form, which allows partners to make referrals online if they prefer, as opposed to the onerous process of printing, completing, scanning, then emailing/faxing a paper form. Once an electronic form is completed, the system immediately triggers the creation of a new record in our database, maps information provided on the form to existing fields, and time stamps the referral. The records are marked with a status that flags them for processing in the order in which it was received and reports are automated, providing an accurate list of pending referrals in real time. This new process made it simple to pass incoming referrals over to the Columbia team on a regular basis, for randomization into the study. Feedback about the new system from partners has been overwhelmingly positive, and over 95 percent of referrals are currently processed through the electronic channel. Now that the initial RCT enrollment period is complete and Columbia is no longer randomizing families, Room to Grow has maintained this system for general enrollment. This improved infrastructure has been well received by frontline staff who helped to conceptualize it, and allows us to maintain a more efficient and equitable system for intake, basing enrollment decisions solely on slot availability and meeting eligibility guidelines.

Using this data, the Columbia team was able to put together an accurate baseline demographic report of study participants compared to a wide sample of recent mothers in New York City. Their findings from the baseline survey show that those who are referred to Room to Grow are very high need, debunking the "creaming myth" once again. Mothers in the Room to Grow study have lower education levels than citywide averages (60 percent have a high school degree or lower, as compared to 52 percent among all recent mothers in New York City); were more likely to live in a shelter (24 percent versus 5 percent); and were more likely to receive government assistance, specifically in SNAP or food stamps (67 percent versus 42 percent), public or cash assistance (36 percent versus 6 percent), WIC (87 percent versus 47 percent), and public housing or government rental assistance (22 percent versus 6 percent). This initial analysis has allowed us to articulate, with increased rigor, the extent to which Room to Grow families experience hardship and has given us firm ground to stand on when speaking to the needs of our client population.

Although these changes created efficiencies that set us up for a smooth transition into the study enrollment period, they were initially met with some resistance from Room to Grow's program team. Our clinical staff is highly protective of program participants and their experience—the warm, personalized environment is a core component of our model and is what differentiates us from many other social services that low-income families encounter. The impact that this new technology might have on relationships, with both families and outside partners, was discussed at length, and feedback about the messaging and style was thoughtfully implemented into the design of the new tools. For example, clinicians stressed the importance of being mobile during a visit—the ability to be on the floor playing with a toddler or sitting in an armchair next to a mother—so being in front of a computer was clearly not an option and tablets were preferred. Also, in the randomization process, Columbia would be the first point of contact for a new family, rather than the clinical team at Room to Grow, creating concerns among our teams that participants may be less willing to enroll. Enrollment scripts were carefully crafted by the Columbia and Room to Grow teams together that both matched the tone and language of the program and also met Institutional Review Board (IRB) requirements. A year and a half into implementing these new systems, there has been no detectable negative impact on participant satisfaction, retention, or enrollment rates. This was a substantial organizational win and a reminder not to assume that thoughtful, well-planned changes in our operations might negatively impact participation, and in fact may even enhance the quality of our interactions with families. Our program model is grounded in the very fact that families are resilient and in many ways masters of managing change in their daily lives—to treat them otherwise is counter to our mission and our work. The tweaks that we made in how we manage the flow of information throughout the program, while certainly a change for our team and program participants, were extremely beneficial. Being pushed out of our comfort zone ultimately helped codify and stream-line our processes, reduce barriers for community partners, and advance Room to Grow as an outcomes-driven, learning organization. These changes will continue to be instrumental as we look to further grow our service reach and expand to other markets while maintaining program quality and fidelity.

While the team worked to establish the operational chops that would allow us to begin enrolling participants in the study, we were simultane-ously doing the legwork to select the measures to compose the partici-pant surveys. Our initial two years of funding from the RWJF allowed us to complete our in-home baseline survey and a follow-up survey when participating children were approximately one year old. This funding cap represented a challenge for our study, as the Room to Grow inter-vention runs for three full years. Though we were committed to fund-raising to extend the timeline, until new funding could be identified, we faced real-world trade-offs in study design, including sample size, methodology (phone survey at year one), and the developmental age of the children at first follow-up, when only certain proximal outcomes could be measured. Therefore we chose to focus on proximal outcome measures that positively predict child development rather than direct assessments of participating children at our first follow-up, which could be better accomplished when a child is older and requires in-person observation. However, the number of possible proximal outcomes—for example, parenting practices, parental health and well-being, material hardships—that positively predict child development were still too numerous to evaluate rigorously within our short, thirty-five-minute year-one phone survey.

Brooks-Gunn challenged us to narrow our focus to a discrete number of outcome domains that we believed most closely aligned with Room to Grow's theory of change for our baseline survey. Initially this was a contentious exercise. Team members—even within Room to Grow—had difficulty aligning on which year-one factors would serve as the best leading indicators. This level of rigorous research challenged Room to Grow to hone our theory of change—that is, clearly articulating our assumptions about the processes through which positive change occurs—including specifying early, intermediate, and long-range outcomes with an understanding of their timing and critical components (Anderson 2006). At that time, we had only recently launched our upgraded internal evaluation structure and had less than six months of internal data to leverage in narrowing down our predicted domains of highest impact. While our data was preliminary, it suggested an important role for outcomes from positive psychology, such as parenting efficacy. Careful qualitative reviews of our curriculum, preliminary internal data, and existing parent satisfaction survey results reinforced our belief that Room to Grow's client-centered philosophy of personalization, dignity, and a strengths-based lens were the most promising pathways for the program's effects. Families volunteered that, while they often felt marginalized or talked down to by staff at other family service agencies, they believed that Room to Grow viewed them as positive agents of change.

These themes were intriguing, and they suggested that—in addition to our original hypothesis about the provision of material support providing an increased value add over parenting education alone—Room to Grow's strengths-based philosophy itself represented an important value add of the program model. Doing the hard work and soul-searching to narrow down our outcome domains to a targeted number, as Brooks-Gunn advised, ended up being one of the most important first steps in establishing a high-functioning practitioner-university partnership and is one of our top recommendations for other teams looking to embark on similar work together. This process surfaced an important lesson: having evidence that a nonprofit is achieving positive impact is not the same as determining *how* it is achieving that impact. If teams default to simply using outcome measures that have commonly been used by others without thoroughly understanding their own unique theory of change, they could easily miss out on valuable and critical learnings. For example, themes of efficacy and empowerment repeatedly surfaced in Room to Grow's internal data, but those domains are still not commonly measured in the broader nonprofit world. If Room to Grow staff members from across the agency had not taken such an active role in the review and development of the baseline survey and volunteered insights from their own preliminary data, the academic team could easily have missed the opportunity to measure these unique proximal outcomes that would later underpin summative outcomes.

Completing Brooks-Gunn's thought exercise became the foundation for revamping Room to Grow's theory of change in a principled manner. We carried forward the initial work the research team had begun in selecting proximal outcomes for the baseline survey by conducting a thorough internal theory of change workshop with all agency staff. Our design process included input from staff at the Harvard Center for the Developing Child based on their Frontiers in Innovation collaboration principles. While the resulting evaluation-aligned theory of change retroactively validated the outcomes and themes we discovered while developing the initial RCT survey, having a solid theory of change at the outset of our research partnership would have saved us significant time and energy.

Even with a targeted set of outcome measures in hand, aligned with our revised theory of change, we found ourselves facing additional challenges in selecting specific questions and measures for the research. Since strengths-based programs are still rare within the social service sector, very few "gold standard" evaluations have included strengths-based outcomes. Many validated assessments are deficits-based—focusing, for example, on reducing instances of child maltreatment instead of increasing instances of positive parenting—meaning their language can be stigmatizing for parents. Given our hypothesis that the strengths-based approach within the Room to Grow program is crucial to our success, we did not want to undercut understanding or further stigmatize study participants by using language within the RCT that reinforced a deficits model.

We undertook an extensive review of the literature and consulted with additional university colleagues and study mentors to ensure that we were measuring strengths-based outcome domains using rigorous and validated measures. For instance, we identified from within previous open-source federally funded Maternal, Infant and Early Childhood

Home Visiting (MIECHV) evaluations of home visiting programs (e.g., the Triple-P Positive Parenting Program) (De Graaf et al. 2008) a set of normed and validated short scales to measure parenting efficacy. We leveraged the qualitative interviews we conducted between the baseline interview and the design of the first follow-up survey to further understand what strengths-based concepts, such as *dignity*, meant to clients, ensuring that the scales we had selected at baseline adequately captured clients' own conceptions of their strengths. Insights from the first round of qualitative interviews suggested that our initial focus on efficacy and other concepts specifically related to *parenting* was too narrow. In response we added questions capturing self-efficacy and additional domains to our year-one survey.

Our partnership in this phase of designing our study taught us that selecting measures for formal evaluation is, ultimately, an exercise in humility. For university partners, it is an exercise in remaining humble to the idea that no one knows how a program works better than its own clients and staff. When we began our study, we were almost uncomfortably in the vanguard, measuring outcome domains that few other projects had considered. However, our work ultimately aligned with emerging trends. Over the past year, we have watched peer organizations begin to confront the stigma inherent to measuring only deficits. Our team members have written and presented, formally and informally, about our study design and how we are working to develop novel capstone outcome measures—including a resilience activation scale—as the next iteration of strengths-based evaluation. For nonprofit partners, research design is an exercise in humility because no single program—including ours—is a silver bullet. We are unlikely to improve all desirable outcome measures equally, despite our best intentions and vision. It is in our best interest to be reflective and discerning about our relative strengths and weaknesses based on honest consideration of the best available program data and a clearly defined theory of change. Nonprofits often undertake evaluation because we want to demonstrate to stable funding sources—public and private—that we are competitive with previously funded programs. If we are truly providing a value add beyond existing validated models, however, then it is unlikely that selecting off-the-shelf outcome measures from the US Health and Human Services Home Visiting Evidence of Effectiveness (HOMEVEE) database or the Institute for Education Science's What Works clearinghouses will fully capture our strengths. We owe it to ourselves and to our partners to develop a nuanced understanding of our own strengths instead of relying solely on the university experts to teach us about our own experiences. Rather combining these field-based and academic perspectives together to create authentic synergy is what will yield a high quality research project and, ideally, leave a nonprofit organization with greater capacity to understand its work and results even in the short term.

Qualitative methods, such as in-depth interviews, are widely used in program evaluation and can be especially useful in understanding how and why an intervention achieves effects. Qualitative data can also inform how a program is implemented, whether or not a program is implemented as intended, and how it is received by their participants (an indicator of sustainability). Qualitative inquiry focuses on participants' experiences in the program and the meaning they attribute to those experiences. Data is typically collected across a limited number of individuals, yet aims for rich descriptions of complex ideas and processes. Our team decided to use qualitative, in addition to quantitative, methods in this project for two main reasons: (1) to inform the design of the data collection surveys, and (2) to explore the "black box" of effects—or, in other words, to try to unpack the specific causes behind any final results.

To capture different experiences, we divided our qualitative research in three groups: clinicians, graduates (clients who completed the three-year program), and participants in the RCT (both in treatment and control groups), and designed different semi-structured interviews for each group. Our three New York City–based clinicians and the RCT participants were interviewed individually, while graduates were interviewed in groups of three to five, based on their preferred language. Our two teams coordinated to contact and facilitate the scheduling of recent program graduates. In selecting participants, it was important to make sure that we captured the experience of diverse cultural backgrounds and that all clinicians' former clients would be represented. We arranged for the clinician and graduate interviews to be held at our family center, a familiar and comfortable space for everyone. The interviews were led by two Columbia research team members, which allowed them to pay full attention to the participants while also ensuring that all questions would be covered during the session. After each interview, the two researchers debriefed and wrote a summary highlighting the main themes, which ultimately became important factors in the design of the surveys used in the study.

In addition to focus groups that pointed us toward key measures, we were able to recruit several client volunteers to pilot the year-one follow-up survey over the phone with us. The duration of the surveys had implications for both budget and researcher time, so this qualitative component was another key feedback loop during the design phase. While it is easy to test the timing of a survey with a colleague, the opportunity to speak with someone in the same demographic as our study participants gave us valuable insight into the practicalities of the project. For example, we got a fairly realistic sense of the survey timing with interruptions from children in the background of calls.

Initially we also had some concerns about how the content and language in our survey might come across to families. Our teams invested significant time and effort editing the terminology in our survey questions and developing guiding language for probing on potentially sensitive or triggering topics (e.g., how we asked about illegal substance use). Keeping our positive, strengths-based approach in mind, we wanted to be thoughtful about language, particularly since the year-one survey was to be administered over the phone. Thankfully, participants in the pilot calls offered honest feedback, giving us a good sense of how the questions landed, addressing our concerns. Our high enrollment consent rate (95 percent) at baseline and the extensive feedback our participants volunteered reinforced that our efforts were fruitful. If a research team genuinely desires to understand how answering their questions makes someone feel and to ensure they are balancing collecting valid evidence with the well-being of participants in a study, then there is no more direct way to do so than to ask pilot participants directly—be prepared to hear "soul-crushing" feedback, though. Moreover, our graduates were eager to contribute to the pilot, and their desire to give back to Room to Grow was clear to the research team, reinforcing the power of collaboration at the heart of community-based research.

Data Collection in Practice

Once the planning and initial design of the study was complete, lessons continued to emerge through the research team's experience administering baseline surveys in the field. Room to Grow's model is center-based, meaning that families travel to us to receive program services. While our curriculum covers home environment and family stability, our clinicians do not see or experience firsthand the challenges that families experience at home. Through the experience of the research team in administering the in-home baseline survey, we gained a deeper understanding of the complex systems that our families must navigate on a day-to-day basis. One of the most onerous challenges our families face, particularly in New York City, is the housing system. While stable housing is often a topic of conversation between clinicians and families during visits, and we anticipated that some of our study participants would be living in temporary housing, we were surprised by the formal percentage—approximately one-third of the pregnant mothers we interviewed were living in a shelter or had lived in one during their pregnancy—most often due to an eviction, job loss, or lack of social support. The complicated layers of the city's shelter system unfolded as Columbia's researchers navigated these cases (Institute for Children, Poverty, and Homelessness 2017). Shelter protocols often required the team to jump through hoops to meet or even talk to participants over the phone. In the simplest of cases, they were required to bring a photo ID and sign a logbook. Most of the time, however, coordination with the main office and the participant was necessary to prove that their services were intended to help the mother and that the visits were in good faith. At domestic violence shelters, where protocols were particularly strict, the research team was often denied access and would have to meet participants offsite. The most difficult cases to coordinate were the ones in which the mothers were not able to leave the shelter, nor were they allowed visitors. In those instances, the mother would coordinate our interview to align with medical appointments, and we would often meet near their healthcare provider's office or in the waiting room.

Shelters that granted access to researchers offered us a glimpse into the typical living conditions of families relying on the public housing system. Poverty is often linked with overcrowded housing, and single-room units push this to the extreme. In one home visit, there was a family living in a single room with three twin beds—two pushed together for mom and dad on one side of the room, one for their young daughter several feet away. This pregnant mother hoped that their housing voucher would come through before she gave birth because the thought of having a family of four, including a five-year-old waking up hourly with a newborn, was just too much. Many shelters across the city operate out of motels or hotels, whether through a designated shelter floor or fully converted into shelter units. This model offered the advantage of most rooms being relatively new, but the implications for food access were troubling. Most mothers had a mini fridge, but no way to properly cook meals. At best, the kitchen in some shelters consisted of a microwave, mini fridge, and a sink, with minimal counter space. Nonperishable items—peanut butter, ramen noodles, and sugary breakfast cereals—were common staples: not the ideal nutritious diet for new or expectant mothers.

The shelter system requirements are often stringent, and there are many pitfalls in maintaining eligibility. For example, a mother who recently gave birth took a job as a caretaker overnight on the weekends, not realizing she was not allowed to spend the night out of the shelter. She first received a warning and was then told that she could no longer stay there. Policies like this often are not clear to participants up front, especially when there is a language barrier. Having to uproot and relocate again significantly compounds challenges, especially when families discover they are expecting a baby. One family had been living in a shelter in the Bronx for two years but, when the mother became pregnant, the shelter moved her and her husband and three children to another location in Queens because they said they were not equipped to house pregnant women. This mother told the research team that the conditions in her original "unequipped" shelter were actually far better than this new shelter, but her main issue with the move was the long commute—the equivalent of four hours a day to take the children to and from their school. On top of that, her entire support network remained in the Bronx. Despite immediately submitting a request to be relocated back to the Bronx, her understanding was that it probably would not be processed until after she gave birth. These stories illuminate the challenges we know that our families face—such as unstable housing situations, food insecurity, overcrowding—but also highlight the feat that families achieve when they consistently attend their quarterly visits to Room to Grow, achieving 90 percent annual retention and attendance markers despite these many challenges (Maternal Infant and Early Childhood Home Visiting Technical Assistance Center 2015).

The poverty researchers on our team spend their time studying the underpinnings of inequality and the hardships that people face. This information often comes from large data sets: the US Census, the New York City Poverty Tracker—studies that are large and anonymous (Garfinkel et al. 2019). While collectively the team has decades of experience in understanding poverty, this study put them in the same room with poverty in a way that most of their previous research had not. Objectivity remained crucial but, at times, ethical boundaries became more difficult, which is where the close collaboration with Room to Grow became indispensable. Some cases were severe and the researchers alone did not have adequate resources; they needed guidance from those who understood the network of services in the communities they were entering. One afternoon, another researcher on our team showed up to conduct an interview in Brownsville, one of the poorest neighborhoods in Brooklyn. The participant quickly ushered her into her bedroom and shut the door. She was young, petite, and eight months pregnant. As she began answering questions about her housing situation and the bedroom she was renting, she revealed that in the preceding weeks her roommate had become aggressive toward her to the point of physical violence. She had reported it to the police, but there were no corresponding support resources. Now she was scared, socially isolated, and pregnant. Knowing this mother was in the control group and would not receive Room to Grow treatment services, our research team felt an ethical obligation to connect her to other supports. They reached out to one of the clinicians at Room to Grow, who had a contact at a domestic violence organization, and were ultimately able to give the study participant a trusted resource. Instances like this one highlight the realities of community-based research—we were in communities that let us in; participants told us and showed us intimate and difficult parts of their lives. In return, we listened and, when appropriate, offered tangible support, preserving both the integrity of our research and our ethics.

Another key component of our research partnership in practice has been our collaboration around retention of study participants. Many participants are balancing motherhood, part-time jobs, classes (whether it be parenting support, legal support, addiction counseling, or personal support), doctor's appointments, and appointments at benefits offices. Additionally, the transient nature of our population means that phone numbers and addresses often change—a challenge that Room to Grow program staff navigate on a daily basis. Our field researchers use "study cells"—iPhones with dedicated phone numbers used to stay connected with participants. Staff members take these phones home and are able to call and text participants with much more ease and flexibility than a standard office landline phone would allow. Oftentimes texting is far more effective for staying in touch than a phone call, since many participants have limited prepaid minutes. Many study participants have reached out voluntarily in between planned touch points with updated information in an effort to stay in contact. These practices have enabled us to be successful in our contact attempts, despite the fact that families can be very difficult to reach by the time they are eligible for the year-one survey. As a tactic to remain in contact prior to our second formal touchpoint at year one, halfway between the baseline and first follow-up, Columbia mails participants a small notepad with a letter reminding them of the follow-up and requesting they reach out to us if any of their contact information has changed. The notepad is embossed with Columbia's logo as well as contact information for the study staff. It is an affordable way to thank our participants for their ongoing participation and to try to revive contact before it is time to complete the next survey. Many of these mail pieces return to sender unopened, prompting us to try to reconnect another way well before participants are due for their follow-up survey. When it comes time for survey follow-up, the team tries to reach our participants by all means available, including phone, email, family/friend contact, Facebook, via referral partners, and through letters mailed by USPS. Reaching treatment participants has proven to be slightly easier, since Room to Grow clinicians are ongoing in contact with families and are able to pass along updated contact information to the research team when needed. For control participants, it is often more difficult to get in touch when contact details change. If phones, addresses, and emails do not work, we have IRB approval to maintain a Facebook business profile and privately search and message participants on social media. We are continuing to consider additional retention strategies as our study continues over time in order to maintain our high retention rates, such as increased incentives for control participants and additional reminders like refrigerator magnets with our contact information.

Messaging and Dissemination

Our mixed-methods research—RCT, auxiliary process evaluations, and qualitative data—are designed to provide empirical evidence of our impact and inform data-driven practice and continuous quality improvement for Room to Grow and, by extension, the wider field of early childhood services. However, Room to Grow's ability to spring-board from that evidence and position itself as an innovative leader in the field depends on more than just validating another "fad" parenting education program. Room to Grow benefits from, and struggles with, its nature as a hybrid program model that draws on elements from multiple fields. On the one hand, hybrid models currently lack any natural "home" in the public funding landscape and can be challenging to convey to policy leaders given that they do not neatly fit into any one funding category or budget line item. Despite this, even in the short term, we are advancing much more than Room to Grow as a discrete program. We are, at heart, making the case for an entirely new philosophy of social service provision—the combination of social supports and material supports through a prevention approach. This philosophy is one that Room to Grow has developed through over twenty years of experience in the field. Ultimately we believe that this combined support approach should be implemented across multiple agencies, disciplines, and cross-sector partnerships well beyond the walls of our current centers.

The Room to Grow message encompasses two critical components that have been largely absent from traditional academic discussions of program effects. The first is that strengths-based programming allows parents to build their own resilience through achieving personalized goals in addition to simply reaching agency-selected targets. The majority of current two-generation program models are still based on the traditional early childhood education (ECE) classroom or around a parenting curriculum that replicates much of the ECE experience in-home. "Wraparound" supports are increasingly provided to parents, but too often take the limited form of screening for referrals to one of a select list of external services, rather than dedicated programming for both parents and children. Room to Grow challenges this traditional approach, centering its services on the parents' experience as much as the child's, with the understanding that by setting parents up for personal success in their child's first few years, they can naturally leverage that success to sustainably support their children's healthy development long-term. The second component is that alleviating material hardship is an integral part of supporting families to sustain positive changes. Low-income parents commonly report feeling caught in a catch-22 when they are taught that they should be doing something—such as reading to their child daily—but still face the daily reality that there is simply no money left for books after providing basic necessities and no time left after working variable shift jobs. Instruction on best practices in parenting without providing a realistic means by which to implement this advice is potentially counterproductive, demoralizing and shaming parents for not engaging when, in truth, they are eager for any means by which to do so. Room to Grow addresses this by providing material resources aligned with its curriculum to offset material hardship and ensure that families have everything they need to act on the knowledge, skills, and confidence they acquire.

Listening to our participants share their stories—and sometimes navigating daily challenges alongside them as we attempt to meet them where they are in homes, shelters, and hospitals—has impacted how we hope to communicate our findings. We have come to recognize that program evaluators are not impartial observers of systemic inequities. The venues and language through which we choose to share our results can help to shape the policy narrative of poverty. We have contributed to progressive academic publications, such as the forthcoming *Art of Resistance* volume, that include direct client voice alongside qualitative analyses, and we present at practitioner and community-inclusive conferences, such as the Robert Wood Johnson Foundation's annual Culture of Health conference and the national Zero to Three convening. Additionally, we have revamped much of the language we use in our publications and grants to elevate the contributions of our families to that of partners instead of just the token "thank you to our participants" comment common at the end of most academic journals. We hope to convey the richness and complexity of their experiences in full, beyond any single data point or anecdote.

Making the case for social change also means taking on an advocacy role and supplementing traditional peer-reviewed publications with thoughtful policy-oriented presentations and op-eds that humanize the experience of poverty. One of our excellent staff researchers, Tonya Pavlenko, has written two experiential op-eds that highlight real case compilations from our study to illustrate the systemic challenges found under the poverty line, such as food insecurity and housing instability. We have also shared key demographics and lessons from our qualitative interviews that highlight the material hardships of our study families with mainstream media reporters and policymakers to advocate for changes that would positively impact families.

Further we have championed social policies that align with Room to Grow's strengths-based and comprehensive support philosophies by participating in citywide collective action initiatives that advance our broader philosophy of social services. Room to Grow provides insight and resources through initiatives such as New York City's Early Years Collaborative and the Boston Opportunity Agenda's Birth Through Eight Collective, where city government officials and thought leaders from healthcare, education, and social services work directly to shape future citywide priorities. We envision a future in which we leverage our experiences in community-based programming and evaluation to act as a peer leader and consultant to agencies seeking to implement these core philosophies in other sectors.

Conclusion

Our collaboration with the Columbia team has taught us the importance of striking a balance between academic rigor and on-the-ground experience, resulting in valuable lessons that we hope will benefit any community program or academic institution looking to forge a similar relationship:

1. Seek honest feedback from stakeholders within and outside of the partnership and establish a culture of open communication and define clear operating norms.

2. Customize outcome metrics to align with the nonprofit's core values, mission, and program model rather than relying solely on commonly used measures.

3. Prioritize participant experience and seek to include meaningful feedback on study design and processes.

4. Leverage research activities to build long-lasting capacity for a nonprofit organization by advancing their internal systems, program rigor, and field knowledge.

At the onset of this project, we could not have imagined the organizational strides that Room to Grow would achieve through engaging in research, advancing operational capacity and program clarity, and achieving greater replicability and even program quality improvement.

It is truly in every nonprofit's best interest to find a research partner that is philosophically aligned, build both a partnership and friendship with them, and find ways to invite them to push at the edges of program quality, consistency, and impact such that the organization comes out the other side better equipped to meet its mission and gains a trusted academic advisor that is always a phone call away. The value add to researchers is not only access to target populations and the opportunity to conduct research but also to understand how the world really works and to advance an evaluator's perception of the value of community engagement and participatory research. In recent months, as we have begun to plan the next stage of our partnership, looking five to ten years into the future, we have been struck by how deeply our research team now understands our work, our strengths, and our challenges. Increasingly, universities are prioritizing the application of their research to drive tangible social change. As this trend continues, it is all the more important to find and forge authentic partnerships and achieve meaningful integration of research and service that enhances diverse perspectives and leaves everyone better for having gained a shared understanding.

References

Anderson, A. 2006. "The Community Builder's Approach to Theory of Change: A Practical Guide to Theory Development." http://www.theoryofchange.org/pdf/TOC_fac_guide.pdf.

Brooks-Gunn, J., and G. J. Duncan. 1997. "The Effects of Poverty on Children." *Future of Children* 7 (2).

Chaudry, A., and C. Wimer. 2016. "Poverty Is Not Just an Indicator: The Relationship between Income, Poverty, and Child Well-Being." *Academic Pediatrics* 16 (3): s23–s29

Citizens' Committee for Children. 2015. "Campaign or Children: NYC's Early Childhood Education System Meet Only a Fraction of the Need." https://www.

cccnewyork.org/wp-content/uploads/2016/06/CampaignforChildren_Child CareNeed_2015.pdf.

De Graaf, I., P. Speetjens, F. Smit, M. De Wolff, and L. Tavecchio. 2008. "Effectiveness of the Triple P Positive Parenting Program on Parenting: A Meta-Analysis." *Family Relations* 57 (5): 553–66.

Flacks, J., and J. R. Boynton-Jarrett. 2018. "Strengths-Based Approaches to Screening Families for Health-Related Social Needs in the Healthcare Setting: Preview of Recommendations." Washington, DC.

Institute for Children, Poverty, and Homelessness. 2017. "On the Map: The Dynamics of Family Homelessness in New York City in 2017." https://www.icphusa.org/reports/map-dynamics-family-homelessness-new-york-city-2017/.

Maternal Infant and Early Childhood Home Visiting Technical Assistance Center. 2015. "MIECHV Issue Brief on Family Enrollment and Engagement." https://mchb.hrsa.gov/sites/default/files/mchb/MaternalChildHealthInitiatives/Home Visiting/tafiles/enrollmentandengagement.pdf.

Substance Abuse and Mental Health Services Administration. 2014. "Trauma-Informed Care in Behavioral Health Services." Treatment Improvement Protocol series 57, HHS publication no. (SMA) 13-4801. https://www.ncbi.nlm.nih.gov/books/NBK207201/.

Wilson-Simmons, Y., Y. Jiang, and Y. Aratani. 2017. "Strong at the Broken Places: The Resiliency of Low-Income Parents." http://www.nccp.org/publications/pdf/text_1177.pdf.

Wimer, C., I. Garfinkel, M. Gelblum, N. Lasala, S. Phillips, Y. Si, J. Teitler, and J. Waldfogel. 2019. *Poverty Tracker: Monitoring Poverty and Well-Being in NYC*. New York: Columbia Population Research Center and Robin Hood.

Yeung, W. J., M. R. Linver, and J. Brooks-Gunn. 2002. "How Money Matters for Young Children's Development: Parental Investment and Family Processes." *Child Development* 73 (6): 1861–79

Chapter 7

Building Strong Partnerships with the Puerto Rico WIC Program for Promoting Healthy Lifestyles in Early Childhood and a Long-Lasting Culture of Health

Maribel Campos
University of Puerto Rico

Cristina Palacios
Florida International University

Alexandra Reyes
Puerto Rico WIC Program

Chapter Context

Maribel Campos: As a pediatrician who specializes in perinatal exposures, I am interested in improving the environment in which our children develop so that they can aspire to and maintain optimal health. However, the genesis of my passion for the field of developmental origins of adult diseases is that I have suffered from obesity since early in life and have also carried the burden of the complications associated with the condition. I have had the benefit of having resources available to address my needs, but most families do not have that advantage. I seek to use my life experiences and knowledge to inform community- and institutional-based practices through collaborative efforts, while acknowledging the power for change where it truly lies: with our children.

Cristina Palacios: As a nutrition researcher, particularly infant nutrition among WIC (Women, Infants, and Children) participants, I was very worried about the quality of dietary patterns of infants in Puerto Rico and how this was affecting their development. This work led to my involvement with the

Puerto Rico WIC program. The WIC program is particularly important in Puerto Rico, as approximately 80 percent of the population participate in this federal program. Because WIC is a community program, it is really accessible to most mothers and children on the island and has a large influence on their nutritional status. I have experienced firsthand the importance of adequate nutrition from birth and how that influenced the health of my children. Therefore I sought to build strong partnerships with the Puerto Rico WIC (PR-WIC) program to promote healthy lifestyles in early childhood and to help create a long-lasting culture of health.

Alexandra Reyes: As a registered dietitian with the Puerto Rico WIC program, my work helps optimize the health and nutritional state of women and children through nutrition and breastfeeding education. I believe that differences in nutritional experiences at critical periods in early life can program a person's development, metabolism, and future health. I learned and witnessed how important early life interventions are, particularly using a system-level approach to address multiple obesity risks factors. The WIC program successfully participated in this community-based project to implement a culture of health in our society. The experience has allowed PR-WIC to align itself with existing efforts and build lasting collaborations.

One of the key elements of the WIC program is to provide a standardized nutritional education curriculum to low-income groups. Puerto Rico has high prevalence of obesity from infancy, and the PR-WIC program is key in helping reduce this major health problem. There are challenges, however, particularly with low participation rates in educational activities. We sought to increase the dissemination of key components of the WIC nutritional education curriculum to empower participants in the development of healthy lifestyle choices through the process of community-based participatory research. PR-WIC was our community partner. The project faced several challenges, including: (1) major changes in the organizational leadership team, which significantly affected our established communication plan and resulted in changes that had an impact on the final project as implemented; (2) major changes within the team, which once again required a shift in the management of the project; and (3) two major hurricanes, which shifted the priorities for a significant amount of time to assist our community partner in other areas during the state of emergency.

Some of the lessons learned were: (1) understanding the problem—a task that took several years of research with PR-WIC participants and staff; (2) adapting to government changes and changes in the PR-WIC leadership team; (3) establishing the community-based participatory research model; (4) merging agendas between the community partner (PR-WIC) and the academic partners; (5) participating in additional training in community-based participatory research to better understand the principles and be able to establish a true partnership with the PR-WIC program; (6) involving the WIC program in the dissemination of results to make sure their voices were heard; (7) recognizing other important stakeholders, such as other health professionals and the technology partners, in addressing the obesity health issue using technology; and (8) building resilience to help the team continue in the face of the different challenges experienced.

Introduction

Childhood obesity is a growing problem with higher prevalence among Hispanics, particularly among Puerto Ricans, and among low-income families and participants of the Women, Infants, and Children (WIC) program. A key element of the WIC program is to provide a standardized nutritional education curriculum, which could help reduce these disparities. However, there are challenges in delivering the educational component in WIC due to low participation rates in Puerto

Rico. Therefore, as part of the Interdisciplinary Research Leaders (IRL) program of the Robert Wood Johnson Foundation, our main goal was to increase the dissemination of key components of the WIC nutritional education curriculum to empower participants in the development of healthy lifestyle choices.

Problem: Obesity Early in Life

Childhood obesity is a growing problem in the United States and worldwide, with 17 percent of US children being obese (Ogden et al. 2015). Obesity in early infancy is also growing in the United States, with 8 percent of infants meeting criteria for obesity (Ogden et al. 2014). Obesity at such an early stage is predictive of obesity later in childhood and into adulthood (Adair 2014). Several studies have shown an association between increased rates of weight gain during the first four to twenty-four months of life and the risk of being overweight during later childhood or early adulthood (Dattilo et al. 2012; Ciampa et al. 2010). It is likely that infants that have rapid weight gain during the first year continue to increase weight above the guidelines thereafter, setting the stage for obesity later in life (Nader et al. 2006, a longitudinal sample of 1042 healthy US children in 10 locations). Born in 1991, their growth reflects the secular trend of increasing overweight/obesity in the population. Height and weight of participating children in the study were measured at 7 time points. We examined odds ratios for overweight and obesity at age 12 years comparing the frequency with which children did versus did not reach specific BMI percentiles in the preschool- and elementary-age periods. To explore the question of whether and when earlier BMI was predictive of weight status at age 12 years, we used logistic regression to obtain the predicted probabilities of being overweight or obese (BMI

> or = 85 percent). The first one thousand days of life (conception to twenty-four months) are crucial for healthy growth and development (Adair 2014). Infant obesity is a serious public health problem worldwide and increases the risk of chronic conditions associated with obesity, such as hypertension, cardiovascular disease, insulin resistance, and metabolic syndrome later in life (Pray 2015).

There is a high degree of disparity in childhood obesity (zero to twelve years), with higher prevalence among Hispanics. Hispanics have one of the highest rates of obesity, 14.8 percent, compared to any other ethnic/racial group—blacks, 8.7 percent; whites, 8.4 percent (Johnson et al. 2013). As reported by the WIC program, a total of 23.7 percent of children one to five years old are overweight or obese in the United States (Johnson et al. 2013). In Puerto Rico the prevalence is even higher, at 33.9 percent (Ratner et al. 2013). This high infant (zero to twelve months) obesity rate may be related to several risk factors—such as early food exposures and inadequate eating practices—such as shorter breastfeeding periods, early introduction of complementary (solid) foods, the addition of cereal and baby food to bottles, high juice and formula intake, and not being able to identify satiety cues (Dattilo et al. 2012; Young, Johnson, and Krebs 2012; Gortmaker et al. 1999; Rennie et al. 2005; Yin et al. 2005; Grote, Theurich, and Koletzko 2012; Gaffney, Kitsantas, and Cheema 2012; Mihrshashi et al. 2011). Infant obesity is also related to low activity and short sleep duration (Dattilo et al. 2012).

The Community Partner

WIC is fundamental in reaching out to low-income pregnant women and their children from birth to five years old, particularly in Puerto Rico, in which >75 percent participate in the program (Betson et al. 2011). This is a community-based nutritional program with the capacity to reach out to the participants' homes and follow the effects of the nutritional and educational interventions throughout early childhood, particularly during the first thousand days of life. Another strong element is that a standardized nutritional education curriculum is provided to the participants. The WIC program recognizes that teaching nutrition education to parents and caregivers is fundamental in preventing childhood obesity. Knowledge about making the right choices is the main approach to promoting a child's health. They also recognize that nutrition education is considered effective in promoting healthy lifestyles when it results in a positive nutrition-related behavior change. In fact, nutrition education is one of the primary functions of the WIC program. It is the only federally funded nutrition assistance program with legislative and regulatory requirements to provide nutrition education (Food and Nutrition Service U. WIC Regulations-7CFR246). WIC's nutrition education goals are: (1) to emphasize the relationship between nutrition, physical activity, and health, with special emphasis on the nutritional needs of participants; and (2) to assist the individual who is at nutritional risk in achieving a positive change in dietary and physical activity habits, resulting in improved nutritional status and in the prevention of nutrition-related problems through optimal use of the WIC supplemental foods and other nutritious foods. During each six-month period, at least two nutrition contacts—individual or groups sessions—are available to all participants and parents/caregivers of child participants.

Challenges Faced by the Community Partner in Preventing Obesity

However, there are challenges in delivering the educational component in the PR-WIC program—for example, a low rate of child retention/

participation, low attendance to group classes, and the traditional education curriculum, mostly face-to-face contacts. In fact, in 2014–15 the rate of participation in face-to-face classes was only 51.4–52.4 percent. Therefore nutritional education is not adjusted and intended to meet participants' changing needs. Based on these results, the PR-WIC program conducted a survey among 872 PR-WIC participants to learn about participants' preferred methods to receive nutrition education, perceived barriers to attending group classes, and motivations or incentives to participate. A total of 44.2 percent reported that the primary barriers for not attending group classes were work and school schedule conflicts; 16.6 percent cited lack of transportation; and 15.1 percent stated lack of childcare. On the other hand, 39 percent stated that the principal motivator for participating in WIC was to receive nutrition education, and 30.4 percent for the food packages (specific group of approved foods "prescribed" for the dietary needs of each WIC participant). Furthermore, 45 percent said their preferred method to receive nutrition education was using technology, such as SMS, smartphone applications, and the internet.

Based on these results, in-depth interviews were conducted with two hundred PR-WIC participants and staff (administrative staff; supervisors; nutritionists; office clerks; and community champions, identified as breastfeeding peer counselors, who are also participants of the program) in nine different clinics in Puerto Rico in October 2016. The results suggested that the alternate method for receiving the nutritional education was the use of a web page, as most have access to the page using their smartphone and use it frequently to get the information they need. Participants also proposed the use of videos, demonstrations, and handouts to enhance the process. We also learned that there are major discrepancies between the messages provided by health professionals and WIC nutritionists in three key areas: (1) breastfeeding practices and support, (2) age of introduction of other foods and beverages, and (3) interpretation of growth charts for diagnosing obesity. These findings suggested the need to restructure the program to ensure nutrition-related behavior change toward healthy lifestyles and to reach out to other health professionals so that parents and caregivers receive consistent messages that result in healthy eating and obesity prevention.

A strategy to address these challenges incorporates different perspectives in order to address them. Therefore, through the process of community-based participatory research, our main goal was to promote healthy lifestyles among children participating in the PR-WIC program and to encourage families to embrace a culture of health in order to prevent early childhood obesity.

The Project

The partners in this current project are the community PR-WIC program, represented by the dietitian Alexandra Reyes from the nutrition division of the program; the academic researchers from the University of Puerto Rico, Dr. Maribel Campos, and Florida International University, Dr. Cristina Palacios; and the Robert Wood Johnson Foundation, through the Interdisciplinary Research Leaders program. Maribel Campos and Cristina Palacios had been working in collaboration with representatives of the PR-WIC program for multiple years before this opportunity arose, which led to the strengthening of such partnership and preparation for this new project.

For this project, we designed four phases to accomplish our goals:

Phase 1: Assist in the development of a web page for delivering the nutritional education to PR-WIC participants and evaluation of this web page through a randomized control trial.

Phase 2: Motivational interviews targeting healthcare professionals to determine their perception of the WIC program and services provided, causes of childhood obesity, barriers to achieving childhood obesity prevention, and readiness/willingness for change in the current care model.

Phase 3: Provide educational activities to bridge the gap regarding evidence-based guidelines and resources available targeting all health professionals involved in childhood obesity prevention.

Phase 4: Change public policy to build all stakeholders' knowledge for childhood obesity prevention.

Opportunities for Improvement and Continuation of Partnerships

The previous work between University of Puerto Rico researchers and the PR-WIC program had leveraged on the experience and expertise of each of its members as well as honoring the common goals that guided the efforts. This commitment has been key to that overarching goal that kept the team moving through the difficult times during this project.

It has been said that the only thing that is constant is change. In applying to the funding opportunity, the WIC coordinator at that time, Alexandra Reyes, was selected to be the representative of the community partner. In joining the team, Reyes made significant contributions to the project's development by sharing the product of her educational nutrition survey as well as being willing to build on the USDA-Food Nutrition Service–funded special project that would enable the development of an educational web page. The findings for this quantitative survey were further confirmed by an exploratory qualitative study performed during our initial phase of the project. This led to our partnership moving toward the development of an educational web page for WIC participants. Reyes's knowledge and experience in nutrition education fueled our interactions with PR-WIC officials at the administrative level while also keeping the pulse on what participants at the clinic level desired. Reyes's capacity to play that role within our project was subsequently compromised. Changes in the organizational leadership led to Reyes's reassignment to clinic supervisor, which, in turn, limited her involvement in the development of our platform. This significant change affected our established communication plan and resulted in changes that had an impact on the final project as implemented. In spite of these changes, our team was able to provide support to our team members and keep our energy and efforts focused on our primary goal: improving the health of WIC participants. The research team was clear that this required working with the community representatives, regardless of who was at the helm, as in the years of collaboration we had worked with different program representatives as they were appointed to administrative positions. Eventually we reached a new communication plan, through which we made sure that Reyes's role and contributions to our project were acknowledged.

Time would prove that additional changes to our established working plan would be required. As professionals we aim to grow, and as academics and mothers this is enhanced by the challenge of keeping the balance between our professional growth and being present while providing the best conditions for our family. What that looks like for each individual is different, but opportunities present themselves and are acted on based on that vision. Cristina Palacios played the role of our managing principal investigator for the purpose of our project. At the time she led the submission of the grant documentation, she was the only tenured faculty from our team. The initial training and first phase of our project had been completed, including the initiation of our web page design. It was then that we learned that Palacios had accepted a position at Florida

International University in order to be close to her family. This once again required a shift in the project's management. As a team, we had to make difficult decisions on how to manage the project's funds, but eventually we agreed on a plan that would best provide for the study's needs. As study activities would continue to take place primarily in Puerto Rico, and data management agreements would be under the University of Puerto Rico, Maribel Campos became the managing investigator for the research funds under that institution. Accommodating for changes in scheduling, availability, and physical distance in our workflow took time. This challenge only added to the hurdles imposed by the change in administration within our community organization. The use of electronic media, chats, email, and deadlines proved essential to keeping the work moving forward. The ongoing support and understanding of the IRL principal investigators and the skill enhancement achieved through workshops and seminars provided by the IRL faculty allowed our work to continue moving forward. In fact, our team was funded to continue this work to implement an additional lifestyle intervention trial funded by the National Institutes of Health.

Nothing could have prepared us for our biggest challenge. We implemented our pilot and participants were being enrolled at selected clinics. Almost three months into the intervention, disaster struck. In September 2017 Puerto Rico was severely impacted by two catastrophic hurricanes: Hurricane Irma and Hurricane Maria. Almost the entire island was without power for many months. Food security became a major issue as most of the goods consumed are imported and all the ports of entry were disabled. Supermarkets had to discard their inventory due to a lack of power and went without being resupplied for extended periods of time. Arrangements were made by our community partner to ensure continuity of services. More than one year after the hurricanes, there were still some clinics that continued to provide services from displaced locations. During this time, we adapted our efforts in assisting our community partner in other areas until power was restored. For example, we assisted in the maintenance of their electronic data management as clinics without internet access or electricity were documenting in paper records. Aware of the implications to our project, we refocused our energy to ensure the best conditions to our community as a whole. This meant assisting our partners in providing the best care possible under extreme conditions, as it was clear that living conditions were not ideal for anyone after the hurricanes. Service providers within the program had to face the demands and desperation of participants while also dealing with their own losses. Therefore, in the spirit of true partnership, we facilitated a self-care workshop for the PR-WIC nutrition staff. We also helped develop the dissemination posters with the information to access the PR-WIC web page. These were then distributed to all PR-WIC clinics. We also facilitated the meetings to get every clinic on board with this web page. This presented an opportunity to facilitate the dissemination of the platform, through workshops and other activities, while supporting and being sensitive to their needs.

As Puerto Rico continues to heal from the devastation wrought by Hurriances Irma and Maria, it has strengthened our community. Our patience and understanding during this period have reinforced our enterprise, our partnership, and our research team. We were able to get all the data needed to evaluate our project, and we are now analyzing it with plans to disseminate our findings at the National WIC Association, a national online WIC network, as representatives of the PR-WIC program.

Lessons Learned

Over the years, we have learned many lessons for establishing long-lasting collaborations with community partners for the promotion of healthy lifestyles in early childhood and a long-lasting culture of health. Some of these lessons are:

1. *Understanding the problem.* Initially an important aspect of establishing our partnership was the implementation of research studies to better understand the problems within the community. For years we conducted several studies to collect data on anthropometrics to quantify the obesity problem, on dietary patterns, including nutrient intake, food groups intake, feeding practices, and diet quality, and on sleep data and physical activity (Palacios et al. 2018; Banna et al. 2017; Sinigaglia et al. 2016; Palacios et al. 2016; Rios et al. 2016; Molina et al. 2016). We also conducted qualitative studies to understand the input of PR-WIC participants and staff to the problem of childhood obesity. Each project provided us with experiences on what worked and was attractive to the participants of the program as interventions to promote health. However, many of these studies were conducted in the academic environment, without much communication and feedback to the WIC program.

2. *Adapting to government changes.* As a rule, we have all followed the dogma of remaining faithful to our purpose and treading the path for those who might not be able to see what led us to it. For the researchers, this was not be the first time they had faced the challenges imposed by a change in government administration, but it was the first time that we felt the impact it had on one of our own, as Reyes was wholeheartedly one of us. Nonetheless we moved forward with our plan, respectfully engaging additional

community partners as they took office. We then understood that the problem that we were challenged to address demanded that we included others to make sure that the community is represented every step of the way. Reyes continued to be honorable and true in spite of the challenges imposed by changes in her role within the program.

3. *Establishing the community-based participatory research model.* As mentioned previously, our team was composed of a community partner (Alexandra Reyes) and two academic researchers (Maribel Campos and Cristina Palacios). As a team, we applied the principles of community-based participatory research in the writing of the proposal to obtain funds from the Robert Wood Johnson Foundation.

4. *Merging agendas.* Before applying for this funding opportunity from the Robert Wood Johnson Foundation, Reyes also submitted a proposal to the USDA Food and Nutrition Services requesting funds to develop an online educational strategy for the PR-WIC program. This proposal was in response to the aforementioned survey conducted in 872 PR-WIC participants, which showed that participants suggested an online tool instead of face-to-face classes to meet the educational requirement from the WIC program. This was confirmed through our qualitative study. Therefore, as both proposals were funded, we joined efforts to accomplish the development of the online educational strategy. This joining of efforts and funds led to the development of a better educational tool.

5. *Participating in additional training in community-based participatory research.* As part of the IRL program, our team participated in several trainings on community-based participatory research. This was fundamental for our work, to understand the principles

by both the community partner and the academic research partners, and be on the same page. Although some might consider it a basic concept, our first challenge was to define: Who is the community? Is it the program in its entirety; is the community defined by program participants? We learned that in order to achieve a translatable intervention we would define the community as the entire WIC program, including its officers, healthcare providers, and participants. We learned how to work in true partnership with the PR-WIC program in order to ensure that all voices were heard.

6. *Involving the WIC program in the dissemination of results.* Another important aspect of our partnership was learning different strategies to communicate findings to a nonacacemic audience. We also involved our community partner in our publications in order to make sure that they were represented in all dissemination efforts. These were memorable opportunities where we reaffirmed our commitment to our community partners and their needs.

7. *Recognizing other important stakeholders.* During our project we identified the need to include other stakeholders, such as other healthcare professionals, to address the obesity health issue. This was confirmed by findings from our formative study, which indicated inconsistencies in recommendations given by WIC nutritionists and pediatricians as one of the sources of confusion of parents and caregivers. We reached out to physician organizations and linked our exploration study with dissemination of evidence-based practices and epidemiological data from our previous studies. Preliminary data show that there is still much to be done before considering a shared care model between WIC and pediatric healthcare providers in our community. Therefore we have continued with our dissemination activities while channeling feedback from healthcare

providers to program officials as needed. Quality-improvement processes demand honest and objective reflection of where we are so that opportunities for improvements can be identified and addressed. Our role is to perform independent research to inform the community and stakeholders of the opportunities while mediating formative interactions between parties. Thus far the dietitian Jeanette Canino, the PR-WIC program director, has participated in multiple major pediatric societies' meetings, and members of our team have presented in various WIC program educational sessions. Furthermore we also identified the need to incorporate another important stakeholder—the technology partners—since our project directly involves the use of technology for promoting healthy lifestyles in early childhood. This was an unforeseen but essential partner that we did not acknowledge as such in the beginning. Study progress and success are contingent on information systems support and timely response to the strategy being developed. Guidance in the development of strategies and the capacity of the platform to function independently are essential components to our partner. Guaranteeing sustainability and capacity to update content over time are also crucial. However, final plans on project priorities and how to address them are determined entirely by the PR-WIC program. We have been afforded the role of consiglieri to ensure compliance with grant objectives, but final approval requires program officials to intervene, which, on occasion, has resulted in delays.

8. *Building resilience*. The challenges experienced helped us to be resilient and to place the needs of the community before our project needs. As the government changed and our community partner was no longer in the position to execute our project, we became

resilient to change and adapted to new partners. We met with the new administration to understand its needs, to show the progress thus far, and to build trust again. Also, as electricity was reestablished in Puerto Rico after Hurricanes Irma and Maria, as a team we questioned ourselves if we should continue with our project. We engaged in conversations with many different groups, including other IRL members, for their feedback and support. However, after several meetings with the PR-WIC program and within our team, we understood that our community partner needed to continue with the original plans. We are continuing in our analysis of how this web page helped with participants' retention, completion of numbers of educational contacts required by the WIC program, and changes in lifestyle behaviors. We have continued to conduct our interviews with healthcare providers in Puerto Rico and hope to be able to complete our plans in training healthcare providers for infant obesity prevention, which requires a tight partnership with the PR-WIC program.

All these experiences have helped us to improve our long-lasting collaboration with the PR-WIC program for the promotion of healthy lifestyles in early childhood and a long-lasting culture of health.

References

Adair, L. S. 2014. "Long-Term Consequences of Nutrition and Growth in Early Childhood and Possible Preventive Interventions." In *International Nutrition: Achieving Millennium Goals and Beyond*, vol. 78, edited by R. E. Black, A. Singhal, and R. Uauy, 111–20. Basel, Switzerland: Karger.

Banna, J., M. Campos, C. Gibby, R. E. Graulau, M. Meléndez, A. Reyes, and C. Palacios. 2017. "Multi-Site Trial Using Short Mobile Messages (SMS) to

Improve Infant Weight in Low-Income Minorities: Development, Implementation, Lessons Learned and Future Applications." *Contemporary Clinical Trials* 62: 56–60.

Betson, D., M. Martinez-Schiferl, L. Giannarelli, and S. Zedlewski. 2012. *National and State-Level Estimates of Eligibility and Program Reach, 2000–2009*. Washington, DC: US Department of Agriculture, Food and Nutrition Service. http://www.urban.org/publications/412482.html.

Ciampa, P. J., D. Kumar, S. L. Barkin, L. M. Sanders, H. S. Yin, E. M. Perrin, and R. Rothman. 2010. "Interventions Aimed at Decreasing Obesity in Children Younger than 2 Years: A Systematic Review." *Archives of Pediatrics & Adolescent Medicine* 164 (12): 1098–1104.

Dattilo, A. M., L. Birch, N. F. Krebs, A. Lake, E. M. Taveras, and J. M. Saavedra. 2012. "Need for Early Interventions in the Prevention of Pediatric Overweight: A Review and Upcoming Directions." *Journal of Obesity*. doi: 10.1155/2012/123023.

Food and Nutrition Service U. WIC Regulations-7CFR246. https://www.ecfr.gov/cgi-bin/text-idx?SID=a42889f84f99d56ec18d77c9b463c613&node=7:4.1.1.1.10&rgn=div5.

Gaffney, K. F., P. Kitsantas, and J. Cheema. 2012. "Clinical Practice Guidelines for Feeding Behaviors and Weight for Age at 12 Months: A Secondary Analysis of the Infant Feeding Practices Study II." *Worldviews on Evidence-Based Nursing* 9 (4): 234–42.

Gortmaker, S. L., K. Peterson, J. Wiecha, A. M. Sobol, S. Dixit, M. K. Fox, and N. Laird. 1999. "Reducing Obesity via a School-Based Interdisciplinary Intervention among Youth: Planet Health." *Archives of Pediatrics & Adolescent Medicine* 153 (4): 409–18.

Grote, V., M. Theurich, and B. Koletzko. 2012. "Do Complementary Feeding Practices Predict the Later Risk of Obesity?" *Current Opinion in Clinical Nutrition & Metabolic Care* 15 (3): 293–97.

Johnson, B., B. Thorn, B. McGill, A. Suchman, M. Mendelson, K. L. Patlan, and P. Connor. 2013. *WIC Participant and Program Characteristics 2012*. Alexandria, VA: USDA Food and Nutrition Service.

Mihrshahi, S., D. Battistutta, A. Magarey, and L. A. Daniels. 2011. "Determinants of Rapid Weight Gain during Infancy: Baseline Fesults from the NOURISH Randomised Controlled Trial." *BMC Pediatrics* 11 (1): 99.

Molina, J., K. Amaro, C. M. Pérez, and C. Palacios. 2016. "Sleep Duration, Sedentary Behaviors, and Physical Activity across Weight Status in Hispanic Toddlers' Participants of the WIC Program." *Journal of Childhood Obesity* 1 (4): 18–30.

Nader, P. R., M. O'Brien, R. Houts, R. Bradley, J. Belsky, R. Crosnoe, and E. J. Susman. 2006. "Identifying Risk for Obesity in Early Childhood." *Pediatrics* 118 (3): e594–e601.

Ogden, C. L., M. D. Carroll, C. D. Fryar, and K. M. Flegal. 2015. *Prevalence of Obesity among Adults and Youth: United States, 2011–2014.* Washington, DC: US Department of Health and Human Services, Centers for Disease Control and Prevention, National Center for Health Statistics.

Ogden, C. L., M. D. Carroll, B. K. Kit, and K. M. Flegal. 2014. "Prevalence of Childhood and Adult Obesity in the United States, 2011–2012." *Jama* 311 (8): 806–14.

Ong, K. K., and R. J. Loos. 2006. "Rapid Infancy Weight Gain and Subsequent Obesity: Systematic Reviews and Hopeful Suggestions." *Acta Paediatrica* 95 (8): 904–08.

Palacios, C., M. Campos, C. Gibby, M. Meléndez, J. E. Lee, and J. Banna. 2018. "Effect of a Multi-Site Trial using Short Message Service (SMS) on Infant Feeding Practices and Weight Gain in Low-Income Minorities." *Journal of the American College of Nutrition* 37 (7): 605–13.

Palacios, C., S. Rivas-Tumanyan, E. J. Santiago-Rodríguez, O. Sinigaglia, E. M. Ríos, M. Campos, and W. Willett. 2017. "A Semi-Quantitative Food Frequency Questionnaire Validated in Hispanic Infants and Toddlers Aged 0 to 24 Months." *Journal of the Academy of Nutrition and Dietetics* 117 (4): 526–35.

Pray, L. A., ed. 2015. *Examining a Developmental Approach to Childhood Obesity: The Fetal and Early Childhood Years: Workshop Summary.* Washington, DC: National Academies Press.

Ratner, R. G., S. A. Durán, L. Garrido, M. Jesús, S. H. Balmaceda, L. H. Jadue, and S. Atalah. 2013. "Impacto de una intervención en alimentación y actividad física sobre la prevalencia de obesidad en escolares." *Nutrición hospitalaria* 28 (5): 1508–14.

Rennie, K. L., M. B. E. Livingstone, J. C. Wells, A. McGloin, W. A. Coward, A. M. Prentice, and S. A. Jebb. 2005. "Association of Physical Activity with Body-Composition Indexes in Children Aged 6–8 y at Varied Risk of Obesity." *American Journal of Clinical Nutrition* 82 (1): 13–20.

Ríos, E. M., O. Sinigaglia, B. Diaz, M. Campos, and C. Palacios. 2016. "Development of a Diet Quality Score for Infants and Toddlers and its Association with Weight." *Journal of Nutritional Health & Food Science* 4 (4): 1–15.

Sinigaglia, O. E., E. M. Ríos, M. Campos, B, Díaz, and C. Palacios. 2016. "Breastfeeding Practices, Timing of Introduction of Complementary Beverages and Foods and Weight Status in Infants and Toddlers Participants of a WIC Clinic in Puerto Rico." *SpringerPlus* 5 (1): 14–37.

Stettler, N., B. S. Zemel, S. Kumanyika, and V. A. Stallings. 2002. "Infant Weight Gain and Childhood Overweight Status in a Multicenter, Cohort Study." *Pediatrics* 109 (2): 194–99.

Whitaker, R. C., J. A. Wright, M. S. Pepe, K. D. Seidel, and W. H. Dietz. 1997. "Predicting Obesity in Young Adulthood from Childhood and Parental Obesity." *New England Journal of Medicine* 337 (13): 869–73.

Yin, Z., J. Hanes Jr., J. B. Moore, P. Humbles, P. Barbeau, and B. Gutin. 2005. "An After-School Physical Activity Program for Obesity Prevention in Children: The Medical College of Georgia FitKid Project." *Evaluation & the Health Professions* 28 (1): 67–89.

Young, B. E., S. L. Johnson, and N. F. Krebs. 2012. "Biological Determinants Linking Infant Weight Gain and Child Obesity: Current Knowledge and Future Directions." *Advances in Nutrition* 3 (5): 675–86.

Chapter 8

In Search of Child Welfare and Child Health Collaboration

Lina Svedin
University of Utah

Tonya Myrup
Utah Division of Child and Family Services

Kristine Campbell
University of Utah, Center for Safe and Health Families, Primary Children's Hospital

Chapter Context

The overarching purpose of this team's research is to improve outcomes for infants who are at increased risk for child abuse and neglect, both in Utah and around the United States. Our team worked on building greater connection and collaboration between child protective services (CPS) and child healthcare providers to strengthen the safety net for these children and families.

Kristine Campbell is a child abuse pediatrician and clinical researcher. Her research focus lies in describing disparities in health risks and health outcomes for children with a history of child welfare involvement and identifying promising practices that may improve these outcomes. She has long recognized that these goals cannot be achieved through any single sector, and was excited by the prospect of collaborative research with the Interdisciplinary Research Leaders (IRL) team.

Tonya Myrup is a licensed clinical social worker and a veteran of child welfare services. She has over twenty years' experience, starting as a CPS caseworker. She worked in several program areas before becoming assistant director for Utah's Division of Child and Family Services. She cares deeply about the families the division serves and is always striving to improve outcomes and increase support to employees. Being aware of the toll that constant reform has on an already taxed organization, she is committed to using evidence-based practices and to support research on pressing organizational needs.

Lina Svedin has studied organizational responses to crises extensively and wanted to see how cooperation between key organizations responding to child abuse could be facilitated and supported. Her work on taboo policy topics also led her to appreciate the policy challenges related to effectively governing responses to child abuse. The need for greater cooperation around a vulnerable population—abused and neglected infants—and a desire to give policymakers information on what works and what does not, drew her to the policy-related aspects of the team's work.

The researcher-practitioner team examined the extent to which state regulation allowed, encouraged, or mandated child welfare agencies to collaborate with other professionals, particularly healthcare professionals, in CPS investigations. The analysis provided concrete examples of policies supportive of collaboration for policymakers interested in changing their states' practices. The team also conducted interviews to shed light on the extent to which the practice of collaboration followed policy on paper and, in the cases it did not, how these two diverged. This assessment of how regulation works in practice provides policymakers with critical information to support the implementation of collaborative policies, by uncovering facilitators and barriers to collaboration, and how to measure its effectiveness.

The team also wanted to design and test a collaborative practice that might overcome known obstacles to collaboration. The practice involved CPS caseworkers and primary healthcare providers whose patients were in open CPS investigation. The team trained CPS supervisors and caseworkers in the collaborative practice and ran the practice, with a control group, for eighteen months to understand how collaboration might impact child health as well as parent perceptions of CPS involvement and primary healthcare interventions. This team took several lessons away from these projects. First, they experienced the promise of interdisciplinary collaboration in the setting of complex societal challenges, such as child abuse and neglect. Second, they came to recognize that personal relationships—much more than formal policies and practice guidelines—are the critical elements of collaborative practice. Finally they learned that changing engrained professional practices and asking workers to build bridges across siloed sectors requires time and trust—and not just good ideas and best intentions.

The Scope of Child Abuse and Neglect in the United States

For more than four decades, the federal government has mandated a response to reports of suspected child abuse or neglect by Child Protective Services (CPS) administered through state child welfare agencies. These policies first emerged from professional recognition of the most severe forms of child physical abuse—cases of Battered Child Syndrome and Shaken Baby Syndrome, with victims killed or permanently disabled as a result of inflicted injuries. In the intervening decades, however, societal definitions of child maltreatment have expanded dramatically and involvement with child welfare agencies today may arise from a multitude of concerns. While cases of severe child physical abuse persist, many more children are referred for neglect of a child's physical or emotional needs, exposure to drugs or alcohol, minor physical injuries concerning for abuse, or family violence and dysfunction. Recent research suggests that one in three US children will be the subject of a CPS investigation for abuse or neglect by their eighteenth birthday; one in eight will be identified as a victim of abuse or neglect.

Regardless of the underlying concerns, CPS involvement with a child is a signal of risk for the health and well-being of that child. Compared to children with no history of CPS involvement, children with this history have lower educational outcomes and employment, increased juvenile delinquency and adult criminal involvement, riskier sexual behaviors and more teen pregnancy, higher rates of mental illness and suicide, chronic illness, and early death. Infants referred to CPS before their first birthday face even more specific risks to health and well-being, including repeated episodes of abuse and neglect, foster care placement, and death due to both inflicted and all-cause injury before five years of age. Ideally CPS involvement for suspected abuse and neglect offers a window of opportunity to provide services and support to children and families that may shift the trajectory of social, emotional, economic, and health outcomes associated with this history of childhood adversity.

Unfortunately research indicates we are not meeting these goals. The intervention of CPS caseworkers is intentionally short-lived, and investigations for suspected child abuse and neglect may close within weeks of the initial report. While some cases result in intensive involvement associated with in-home services or foster care placement, many others experience little to no involvement with child welfare caseworkers following case closure. Families may be left with new insight or anxiety related to parenting, yet unsure where to turn for ongoing support and resources. Risk factors for child abuse or neglect—such as substance abuse or intimate partner violence—may be hidden from caseworkers and remain unaddressed during the course of a CPS investigation. Even when CPS caseworkers can fully engage with families, identify household risks, and make referrals to needed resources, their time-limited efforts are rarely shared outside of the strictly regulated silos of the child welfare agency. Real and perceived stigma related to CPS involvement—an experience shared by one in three children in the United States—has restricted the collaboration between the many professionals dedicated to improving the health, safety, and well-being of children.

Interdisciplinary Teaming to Create a Culture of Health in Child Welfare Practice

Frustrated with the lost opportunity to address social determinants of health and childhood adversities offered by the moment of CPS involvement with a family, an informal group of academic researchers, community practitioners, and state agency leaders began to form in the fall of 2015. Discussions in this group centered on a need to prioritize health and well-being in child welfare practices, creating secure safety nets to provide longitudinal support to children and families even after CPS case closure. Interprofessional collaboration and cooperation were rapidly identified as critical resources needed to create a culture of health in the social, medical, and legal responses to suspected child abuse or neglect in Utah. The team research presented in this chapter grew from the interdisciplinary collaboration of three co-investigators involved in these early discussions: Lina Svedin, a policy researcher and university educator with a long-standing interest in promoting collaboration under adverse circumstances and policymaking in the context of social stigma; Tonya Myrup, assistant director of Utah's Division of Child and Family Services (DCFS) with experience in CPS casework at all levels; and Kristine Campbell, a clinical researcher and practicing pediatrician specializing in the evaluation of and response to cases of child abuse and neglect.

This interdisciplinary team came together with a shared goal of improving interprofessional collaborations for Utah infants suspected of being abused and neglected. Fortunate enough to receive funding and training offered by the Robert Wood Johnson Foundation's Interdisciplinary Research Leaders (IRL) program, the co-investigators explored barriers to, facilitators of, and opportunities for innovative collaboration in a series of three linked studies. The first study centered on understanding how and to what extent states around the United States allow or mandate collaboration between CPS and other professional groups, and how the regulatory framework influences on-the-ground collaboration experienced by CPS caseworkers and pediatricians. In the second study, the team planned to examine and compare the implementation of a CPS collaborative practice policy to the experiences other states have had obstacles to and facilitators of interprofessional collaboration. For the third study, the team designed a new child welfare practice intended to improve collaboration between CPS caseworkers and primary healthcare providers of infants with a CPS investigation for suspected abuse or neglect. This new practice was piloted in a randomized controlled trial within two DCFS regions in Utah. This new innovative practice was designed to expand collaboration between child welfare and child healthcare professionals, to improve family perceptions of child welfare and child healthcare involvement, and to improve health-related quality of life for infants with a history of suspected abuse or neglect.

Barriers to Cross-Sector Collaboration in Child Welfare

In 2016 the Commission to Eliminate Child Abuse and Neglect Fatalities noted the current social response to suspected child abuse or neglect "relies primarily on a single government agency to intervene with families who face complex and intersecting challenges." While the burden of child protection lies on the shoulders of child welfare agencies, opportunities for collaborative practices exist. Referral for suspected child abuse or neglect may trigger a response from multiple sectors in the community, including professionals from child welfare, child healthcare, law enforcement, and court systems. In theory this cross-sector response offers the opportunity to address the high social risks and limited resources present in many families involved with child welfare due to suspected abuse or neglect. Unfortunately real and perceived mandates for each of these actors may work at cross purposes in cases of suspected abuse or neglect. Law enforcement officers and attorneys leading investigations into the criminal prosecution of a parent accused of child abuse and neglect may reduce the willingness of that parent to engage in service plans and therapeutic interventions developed by a child welfare caseworker. Medical providers may disagree with CPS decision-making and side with a slighted family in the absence of information from the agency. Medical providers may be unable to provide needed support to struggling families doing their best to access resources recommended by CPS. These points in the system then end up working, in reality, at cross-purposes. As a result of system parts working at cross purposes, the child and the family at the center in this situation may be left with poor outcomes and mistrust in a response system that does not appear to serve the child's interests well. To achieve the kind of cooperation among system representatives and the families involved that would produce positive results the team hypothesized would include sharing information, asking for concerns, and sharing assessments from across the system. This could minimize the risk that actions by one part of the system undermine the efforts of other parts, by coordinating actions taken by different representatives. This type of collaboration could also minimize the number of interactions the family needs to have with the system and reduce duplicate information gathering from families in these situations. There is a need for cross-sector coordination and, to the extent possible, collaboration, in order to create a comprehensive and effective system-level response to a family facing significant problems.

Child welfare is a heavily regulated area of social policy. It is also heavily politicized, with values and processes that child welfare is charged with upholding, including judgment calls individual child protective caseworkers need to make, strongly reflecting the conservative or liberal leanings of state lawmakers. Sometimes the political charge that child welfare work creates translates into frequent policy shifts for child welfare agencies, and sometimes into definitions of harm, risk, and child abuse that do not completely overlap with the definitions and assessments other professional groups use. Understanding the differences in definitions and values sets other parts in the systems are using and prioritizing for their work then becomes imperative for effective interprofessional communication aimed at keeping children and families safe.

Political undertones aside, child welfare across the United States tends to suffer from inadequate funding. Faced with high demands for services, grueling work, and low wages, many child welfare agencies have high caseloads per caseworker and high turnover rates among caseworkers. This turnover challenges collaboration in terms of changing faces in collaborative settings, accumulated knowledge of how the system works being lost, and a subsequent power differential in collaborative settings between more established professionals and child protective services caseworkers who are new on the job.

The potential for adopting laws that eliminate obstacles and support the kinds of system-level collaboration child abuse and neglect seem to warrant is good because social policy matters, such as child protection and child welfare, are, to a significant extent, regulated at the state level. Whether or not states capitalize on this opportunity was an empirical question we wanted to investigate.

Study 1

We were also curious about where in the United States child welfare agencies were doing collaboration well, and with whom they were then collaborating. Were there best-practice states that could serve as a guiding light in terms of how to structure collaboration between the different points in the system that interact with at-risk families? Did state law make this collaboration possible? Did state law seem to mostly facilitate or hinder collaboration? To what extent did these highly collaborative child welfare agencies need laws and policy to make interprofessional collaboration happen successfully?

Study 2

We also wondered to what extent individual states, such as Utah, are like or different from other states when it comes to the conditions that facilitate or hinder collaboration around children at risk of abuse and neglect. We wanted to see if collaboration as a system response around a child was facing unique conditions or if it was subject to the facilitators and constraints we had identified in other states. We decided, as a natural follow-up study to our nationwide scan of laws and policies regulating CPS's collaboration with other professionals and these state professionals' experience working under these policies, to examine Utah's implementation of a collaborative policy since 2016 and compare the policy content and child welfare professionals' and healthcare professionals' experiences working under this collaborative policy.

Study 3

As a positive step forward, toward greater collaboration around at-risk Utah children, we also decided to pilot a new collaborative practice between child welfare and child healthcare professionals in a true randomized controlled trial. Our goal was to see if we could link a CPS investigation, which is necessarily short in duration and narrow in scope, to a medical home, which is comprehensive and long-term in its interaction with and support of families who may have a lot of needs. Our pilot focused on infants referred to CPS because infants are a high-risk group in terms of abuse and neglect with disproportionately poor health outcomes. We thought if CPS caseworkers could strengthen the link between infants, their caregivers, and the baby's primary healthcare provider, these infants could see better health outcomes over time from the point of the investigation. The collaborative practice involved having the CPS worker communicate with the healthcare provider about their involvement and exchange information about potential social risks and health and developmental concerns. CPS would also educate caregivers about the supportive functions a family-centered medical home can provide.

Identifying Community Stakeholders around an At-Risk Infant

The first step in the team's formation was to get the community partner, DCFS, interested in pursuing this research collaboration. The team was fortunate in finding an advocate in the DCFS director, known for his willingness to partner and collaborate with outside agencies. He was quickly sold on the research idea and asked Tonya Myrup to take the lead role in representing DCFS. Myrup recognized the potential burden placed on CPS caseworkers by the proposed research. While Myrup, in general, was supportive of collaborative work, her role in the agency included ensuring workers were not overburdened by new assignments and duties as this may take them away from precious time with families. As the project required additional tasks for CPS workers, Myrup was reticent at first. However, once she learned that if this piloted practice was effective, it could build capacity within the workforce by creating better outcomes for the infants involved, she became committed to making this a solid quality improvement pilot.

Once DCFS had signed on to the value of creating an interdisciplinary researcher and community partner research team, the next challenge was to clearly define the "community" in this project. From a child welfare perspective, Myrup defined the primary community for engagement as the frontline CPS caseworkers who serve children and families coming to the attention of DCFS. Myrup's conceptualization helped the team realize CPS caseworkers were the immediate community this research would engage. While improving outcomes for children and families remained the primary impact objective of the projects, effective engagement with caseworkers was critical and necessary to achieve this objective. The collaborative practice intervention was developed to honor and respect parent preference, yet was delivered to parents through the professional CPS community.

Engagement with CPS caseworkers alone was insufficient. The societal response to suspected child abuse and neglect includes a wide range of community and professional stakeholders. Among them are law enforcement, educators, judges, parental defense attorneys, state attorneys, and healthcare providers. Many goals for CPS intervention for child abuse and neglect across these stakeholder groups are shared, although prioritization of these goals may be different. In some cases, stakeholder goals may be at odds with one another. The team quickly recognized the need to engage the many individuals and agencies involved and invested in the outcomes of these cases for the success of the project.

In Utah, specifically, the number of actors involved in helping the child welfare system achieve quality outcomes grows exponentially if one looks past this first prominent group. One way to envision the sheer number of stakeholders around children at risk of abuse and neglect is to think of a daisy, with every petal around the child in the center representing a different agency, set of professionals, community groups and organizations, along with the child's family, friends, and educators. Further complicating the operationalization of community and concept of key stakeholders in this research was the fact that the state of Utah had been subject to a class action lawsuit over outcomes in its foster care system in the early 1990s.[1]

As a consequence of the lawsuit, the list of stakeholders who have say or input into the activities and performance of Utah DCFS is substantial. Although this is an important part of a healthy and innovative system, it can also lead to the development of solutions, and new programs add

---

1. This lawsuit resulted in a rigorous settlement agreement, much of which was incorporated into the law that governs the agency. This included the creation of several actively involved oversight agencies. The office of Child Protection Ombudsman was created to investigate complaints against Utah DCFS and a new office within the Department of Human Services, the Office of Services Review, was created. These oversight bodies were charged with conducting robust qualitative and quantitative reviews of the agency's work, and the agency was charged with meeting high standards. Twenty-four years later, Utah DCFS was still reporting annually (at a minimum) to the Child Welfare Legislative Oversight Committee and Social Services Appropriations on how it was performing with regard to these high standards. The creation of the Child Fatality Review Committee was also a result of the lawsuit, and this committee was charged with making recommendations about changes to the Utah DCFS organization and its practices. Finally the Child Welfare Improvement Council was also established to help guide Utah DCFS on policy and practice issues to ensure quality outcomes.

disproportionately to the workload of an already overworked front line. When looked at myopically, adding a few extra duties to a CPS caseworker may seem insignificant. When looking at all of the stakeholders who have influence over the agency and its practice, however, it is important to realize each new or added practice, while adding positive solutions, ultimately falls on the shoulders of the frontline caseworkers.

Challenges and Successes in Engaging with Community Stakeholders

The team also made explicit efforts to engage the most important stakeholders in these childen's lives—the caregivers. Mothers who had previously been involved with child welfare were identified and invited to a focus group. This process went well, and the mothers were deeply engaged and open in the process. They discussed some of the challenges and specific interventions that supported or did not support their success. They supported having CPS caseworkers speak with their child's primary care physician. One mother indicated she would have appreciated this, as she told her CPS caseworker everything and he knew as much about her as anyone. This helped confirm that we were moving in the right direction. The goal is that when DCFS is involved, the right interventions and services are provided at the right intensity to help secure the parents' success and prevent the family from returning to DCFS in a new investigation. Formal ongoing supports, such as physicians, might be a big part of a family's continued success. The mothers in the focus group also talked about how important the caseworker was. One mother attributed her success to the fact that her caseworker believed in her. This may have been the first in what the team came to experience as an ongoing theme regarding the importance of relationships.

The research team's ongoing engagement with mothers who had been involved in a CPS investigation was not as strong as it could have been. The team garnered some very helpful information and feedback but were not sure what more to pursue beyond this. In retrospect the team could have re-engaged these mothers again to provide an update on the progress in implementing processes and explore ways caseworkers could build trusting relationships that would encourage the caregivers to sign a release of information form.

Organizational changes presented barriers as well. During the study, unbeknownst to the research team, the release of information form had been changed by the legal department to require a notary signature. This was identified as a deterrent to caregivers and their willingness to sign a release form. This prompted engagement with the DCFS legal team in an effort to streamline the release process for this particular practice.

The team was continuously engaged with DCFS's attorney to navigate the tricky legal waters regarding the release of information. The team needed clarity and assistance on developing a release that would ensure that the confidentiality rights of the parent and child were respected in an understandable language. The traditional DCFS release of information form is complicated, and the research team wanted to make the process as easy as possible for both the worker and family. Most importantly, the team remained acutely aware of the difference in power between DCFS and the caregivers involved in a case. It would have been easy to obtain a release and, in reality, one may not even legally have been required, but this additional effort was taken in the name of collaboration and respect for the family. True collaboration with a family, the team was convinced, should not involve coercion.

One of the greatest challenges for the team turned out to be effective and ongoing engagement with the CPS caseworkers. It would be very

easy and even understandable for caseworkers to put little effort into
the new practice the team was piloting. The team realized that effective
engagement with caseworkers and their supervisors would be essential
to garnering buy-in and commitment to the proposed practice pilot.
During the course of the study, turnover of caseworkers in the Utah CPS
regions the team worked with rose to approximately 30 percent. What
this meant for the research team was an almost continuous training effort
and outreach to caseworkers and supervisors, as new caseworkers came
on board, to maintain focus and fidelity to the practice. This challenge
was compounded by the simple fact that workers are very busy, and the
flow of qualifying cases cannot be managed. The caseworkers the team
worked with already carry high caseloads and sometimes went several
weeks or months without cases that qualified for the pilot practice. For
the CPS caseworkers, this meant an intentional effort would be required
on their part to remember and implement the practice as trained when,
intermittently, a qualified case came up.

To maintain a connection to the workers, monthly newsletters created
by the research team were sent to the caseworkers. The newsletters
contained interesting information as well as a natural opportunity for a
reminder to do the practice and ask questions if needed. The newsletter
also had the unanticipated benefit of forcing the research team to stay
on top of the list of CPS caseworkers currently enrolled in the collaborative effort group. Each month Tonya Myrup had to check and compare
the list of caseworkers currently involved in the pilot practice to the list
that last month's email went to, in order to delete the email addresses of
workers who had quit or transferred somewhere else in the agency in the
last month.

The research team also had to attend to regional differences. Two of
the five DCFS regions were engaged in the pilot practice, and the regions

presented stark differences in organizational cultures and contexts. One region was known by DCFS administrators to be more compliant with new policies being implemented but had less experienced staff with some of the highest turnover rates in the state. The second region was known to frequently question new practices and approaches. This region's culture was to ultimately embrace something new, but it needed more contextualization and to know the reasons why decisions are made before fully engaging with a new process. This region had more experienced CPS caseworkers and tended to hold strong opinions about the work the agency does. This required the research team to adopt slightly different approaches when engaging the caseworkers and their supervisors.

The research team took advantage of a site visit by a representative from the program that funded the research to reach out again to case-workers. The team invited CPS caseworkers in the study to lunch and a conversation about the project, to show the site visitor the work the team was doing to support continuous engagement with caseworkers and their supervisors. Unfortunately the timing was poor as the proposed lunch had to be scheduled right before a holiday and the team knew the turnout would not be ideal—yet the team ended up pleasantly surprised. The lunch had a great showing, with two supervisors and about ten case-workers attending. The partners engaged in the pilot had the chance to share stories and insights into the practice, as well as what was working and what was not. At this lunch the assembled caseworkers and supervi-sors provided some good suggestions to help workers support each other in implementing the practice and ensuring it is done in the way intended.

Factors that facilitated the engagement with caseworkers and super-visors was a previous relationship with either Campbell or Myrup. Those who had an existing relationship with either women were more likely to buy into the process faster and with more enthusiasm. With Myrup, there was the issue of her role in the research team as opposed to her role in the agency. Even though these different roles were explained and separated in each training of caseworkers, the team realized that Myrup filling several important roles simultaneously was confounding for some and likely influenced some of them. Those who viewed Myrup's position as having influence over their own work life and the shaping of organizational practice, the team understood may have been more likely to engage, comply, and be helpful.

Becoming an Interdisciplinary Research Team

Interdisciplinary team-based research is hard but worth it. It requires significant personal efforts to understand, to communicate and be understood, to balance personal preferences with team or research topic needs, to see where others may know best and where you are able to contribute but without taking over. It requires respect, vulnerability, an open mind to learn from others, to listen and to adjust to the group rather than go it alone, even when you think you know best. It also takes a lot of coordination and working out logistics—something that community partners in particular, but researchers too—typically do not have a lot of time for. Equally true is the fact that through interdisciplinary team research we can get to knowledge, understanding, and a depth and width of explanation that is not otherwise possible. Which is precisely why interdisciplinary community-engaged research is up to the task of tackling the most complex and persistent health-related issues we face. The research quality and value that can be achieved through team research is worth the personal effort and institutional wrestling required to do it.

Recognizing that team-based research across disciplines or spheres is challenging, there are a few things this team did that helped them grow and strengthen at the same time as they developed their research plan. In this work, each team member came to the complex problem of child abuse armed with their own set experiences and perspectives, each with limited insight into the experiences and perspectives of their teammates. This reality forced the intentional development of a collaborative interdisciplinary team in parallel with the interdisciplinary research on child welfare collaboration described earlier. Traditional models of interdisciplinary research may highlight long-term collaborations across disciplines and practices. The reality, however, is such that interdisciplinary teams may form quickly in response to funding opportunities, policy requirements, or chance. As fellows with the RWJF Interdisciplinary Research Leaders program, this team's growth as an interdisciplinary research team was intentional and shaped key decisions in their research.

Interdisciplinary collaboration grows from respect for the other team members' expertise, experience, and contribution to the team. This interdisciplinary team bridges a number of divides—academic research and practice as well as working across substantive areas of expertise—child welfare service and social work, pediatric clinical work and medical research, and public policy research and teaching and training. In order to gain a better understanding of each other's worlds, working conditions, and values, and to foster trust and respect for each other's different perspectives, each team member made a conscious effort to shadow or participate in another team member's work early on in the research process.

Child protection and child welfare are complex policy areas, and the realities facing caseworkers, supervisors, and child welfare administrators may be difficult to grasp for an outsider. Campbell and Myrup both have ample experience in the child welfare world. As a way to better understand these realities and the organizational learning processes that have been instituted to guarantee continuous improvement, accountability, and transparency, Lina Svedin, who had limited experience with child welfare, was invited to walk in Myrup's world for two full days early on in this team's research process.

Lina Svedin was trained as an outside reviewer and participated in a two-day annual qualitative case review process with Utah's Division of Child and Family Services. Through this process she learned all the best practices caseworkers and the division aim to apply in cases of child welfare investigations, and she got to review the quality of the work in one case together with a seasoned child welfare professional, including interviewing as many of the stakeholders involved in the case as possible. This included the caseworker originally assigned to the case; the caseworker's supervisor; interacting with and—if old enough—interviewing the child in question to assess well-being and development; interviewing the child's caretakers at the time of review; speaking with the guardian ad litem, the law enforcement officer who had worked on the case, the prosecutor involved, and a therapist who had worked with the child's mother. Svedin also visited the jail where the child's biological parent(s) were housed to interview them about their experience with CPS in this case. She then had to present the case review and assessment in a larger forum that discussed the reviews of all selected review cases for that year in the region and craft a report for the continuous improvement process. Svedin found this experience to be especially enlightening, as it brought into clear view the realities children and families face, the challenges of case management, and how the agency is constantly trying to make sure its clients get the best support and service it can provide.

Svedin was also able to keep these vivid and tangible experiences from the quality-review process as reference points when discussing the organizational processes and levels of organization in states' child welfare systems later on in trainings and interviews involved in this project.

While the fact that Svedin was the team member who did not have a strong connection to child welfare services or child abuse and neglect pediatrics could have become a source of possible contention and questioning in trainings and stakeholder interviews, the team developed some strong ways of legitimizing Svedin's credentials, and her people skills bridged her gaps in knowledge most of the way. In trainings with CPS caseworkers for the randomized controlled trial, the trainings started by emphasizing that this was a genuine team research effort. Myrup as the community partner in particular emphasized and explained why she wanted to be part of this team, what she thought it would bring to the agency, and how the research fits into already established priorities and practices the agency has. This established the team as a valuable and legitimate group, and the work they were going to do with the caseworkers as important. The remainder of the challenge was to make sure caseworkers understood why they were being asked to do more than their already taxing workload—the team realized this was a significant ask, and this research could not be done without the caseworkers' active lead each step of the way. Svedin's job of training them how to do the specific intervention then became, in essence, a "let me make this as easy and least taxing as possible" exercise, where she was setting them up to succeed with the least discomfort and additional effort possible, and with as much clarity of process as possible.

With regard to the phone interviews the team pursued, Svedin's authority came from being a professor at the university, doing policy implementation research, and having Institutional Review Board clearance to help legitimate the specific research questions. Emphasizing the desire to learn from other states to make Utah's system work better also resonated with many in the pediatric field who find themselves frustrated and challenged by interprofessional collaborations and interactions in their own day-to-day lives. That frustration with and some pride in when those organizational and individual hurdles to coordination were overcome helped set a collaborative tone to interviews, and Svedin tried to overcome gaps in knowledge by being an active listener and not assuming she knew these professionals' reality.

In order to gain greater understanding of the realities that Svedin operates in—graduate education in public administration and public policy as well as research from a social and behavioral science perspective and tradition rather than medical sciences—Campbell was invited to present to and interact with students interested in public policy or working on program evaluation. Campbell presented her research questions and the research approach she wanted to take in a risk-and-harm assessment project she was working on at an interdisciplinary policy at the podium forum, organized by the public affairs master's programs Svedin directs. The questions the students attending the forum asked were not the questions she expected, and there was far less criticism of her methods than perhaps she would have gotten from a more medically oriented audience.

Campbell also had a chance to share the practical and ethical challenges of implementing experimental designs, including randomized controlled trials, in the context of welfare programs with students enrolled in an executive education course on program evaluation for mid-career public and nonprofit administrators. Her interaction with these students, the setting, and the educational format served as an example of interdisciplinary research training. The students were able to hear Campbell's practical research experiences and integrate this into the formal research training being provided through this coursework. Conversely, Campbell had the opportunity to engage with professional-level students with practical experience with program implementation in the public sphere.

Another aspect that has been an important point of growth for this interdisciplinary team has been to understand the language undergirding the disciplines and spheres of practice the other team members operate in. As an extension of that deeper understanding, each team member has needed to stretch to learn how to best engage and communicate with the audiences each team member brought to the table. Some of the audience that the research brought to the table, none of the team members were particularly comfortable and well-equipped to talk to. One example of this was the caregiver with prior involvement with CPS, whom the team wanted to ask for feedback on the research design. However, they approached this challenge together as a team, were supportive of each other's clumsy efforts, and were forgiving of mistakes and miscommunications.

Going into the caregiver feedback session, for example, the team had a shared understanding of the value of parent feedback on the study being proposed and of what some of the components of the research the team needed to solicit feedback on. However, none of the team members knew how the invited caregivers were going to react to the proposed study, the team, what they were being asked to provide input on, or really how they were going to elicit honest feedback. Because many caregivers who have been investigated by CPS do not look back on that episode in their lives with positive memories, it was important to establish trust and to communicate a genuine desire to make the research experience something that would be the least offensive and most helpful to the families under investigation.

Each member of the research team tried to contribute to this conversation the best way they could. Campbell provided a quiet setting with a beautiful view for the meeting. She ordered large quantities of high-quality food, with the specific idea there would be too much food and the participating caregivers would be encouraged to take the extra food home to share with their families. Myrup had prepared Svedin and Campbell on what the process of CPS investigation looks like and may have meant for the caregivers coming to provide feedback. Because she was very aware of the power position CPS and DCFS had played in these caregivers' lives, Myrup sat back and played a purposefully subdued role, trying to minimize any perceived power differential or intrusive perception associated with the division she represents. Svedin took on the role of facilitator of the conversation, making sure to be relatable and genuine, asking honest questions about experience and encounters these caregivers had, and that Svedin was something of a novice about. Being a social science researcher with lots of facilitative experience, the team let Svedin ask questions that were grounded in an honest desire to learn more about caregivers' experiences and how the research process proposed could be made the least intrusive and possibly beneficial to caregivers who were being asked to participate.

The results of the conversation and the key pieces of insight the caregivers provided enhanced the team's belief that they each brought strengths to the research being done, and these strengths could be leveraged at different points in the research process to move the team forward. Being respectful, caring, and supportive of each other's values, strengths, and areas of expertise have also been an important part in creating buy-in for team-based research and trust within the team. Team-based research is not easy—it takes a lot of time, willingness to be unsettled and out of your comfort zone, to be vulnerable, and to be willing to learn from others. This is why seeing that the research is stronger because of what each member brings becomes so important to overcoming the natural tendency to want to do things an easier way; by yourself, the way you like to do it, or to not pursue the research topic at all.

Another example of creating team buy-in and supporting what is important to one another was that the team rolled into its research right as the state legislative session started up. Several bills were on the docket that would have profound implications for DCFS's work, and the health and well-being of children in the state in general. Myrup, at the time serving as the acting director of the state's welfare system, was intensely aware of these proposed bills but limited in her ability to comment as a researcher and engaged citizen, having been assigned a very official role in the process. Myrup's dual role as a research team member brought the proposed bills to Campbell and Svedin's attention much more readily, and they both decided to attend the hearings regarding the proposed bills and publicly comment in the forum in order to improve the design of the proposed bills.

Another example is that as the team started accumulating research findings, they were invited to do a state-of-the-art presentation at the National Ray Helfer Society's annual conference. This is the premier conference for child abuse pediatricians in the world, and an exclusive society Campbell and her peers are very actively involved in. Presenting at the conference was very much a five-day walk in Campbell's shoes for Svedin and Myrup. Svedin was very comfortable with the presentation component of the conference, having spent a lot of time teaching professionals, but was completely blown away by the content discussed at other sessions and the seemingly cavalier or jovial tone of the conversations. Myrup was quite comfortable with most of the conference's content due to her prior experience as a child abuse investigation caseworker, supervisor, and now agency leader. Myrup and Campbell were much more hesitant and nervous than Svedin about presenting only partially completed research, generalizing trends in the findings, and inviting participation and input from such a distinguished audience of experts.

Focusing on each team member's strength, the team managed to host this state-of-the-art presentation with a lot of audience participation and positive feedback, which raised the profile of the work in the eyes of this stakeholder audience.

Closing in on the second year of the team's research project, they had a chance to hold an interactive workshop around their work at an annual conference organized by Utah's Children's Justice Center. The conference attendees were child welfare caseworkers, supervisors, and administrators; law enforcement officers; prosecutors; child advocates; and forensic interviewers from across the state. This was Myrup's home turf, and the team set out to try to communicate in an interactive way with her colleagues and collaborating partners. The workshop was surprisingly well attended, and as soon as participants were encouraged to participate, they enthusiastically shared their experiences. The team received valuable insights on their research from other states and what conditions looked like and experiences were across Utah from different professional representatives working on child and family safety issues. Audience participation was so energetic that the team only got through half of its presentation, but left assured that the workshop had been valuable both for audience members and the team itself.

Fruits of our Engagement Effort

The learning the individual team members, and the team as a unit, experienced performing this research was significant. It has paid off in a number of ways, including spurring a number of long-term collaborations and efforts at funding further research and practice. Campbell and Myrup began to make subtle changes in clinical and administrative work in response to preliminary findings that highlighted the critical role of relationships and trust in effective interprofessional collaboration in cases of child abuse and neglect. Campbell had experiences with CPS caseworkers commenting on a need to reach out to primary care providers and pediatricians describing a phone call received from a CPS caseworker about a child in their practices.

Well before the funding of this project, representatives from the wider group of stakeholders had started meeting semiregularly in response to the Robert Wood Johnson Foundation framework for a culture of health. Many of the themes present in the team's research grew from this dedicated collection of practitioners and researchers. These gatherings became more formalized and consistent as the group transitioned to become the community advisory board for the team's community-engaged research. The research team continued to draw on this community advisory board throughout their research project. Several new research proposals have risen from the relationships growing out of this group. Collaborative efforts around education, advocacy, and practice continue to develop. Several of these collaborative efforts cross practice and academia, and center on continuing to learn about and problem-solving pressing health issues and institutional responses to those issues in Utah.

One of the larger projects that rose out of the advisory committee for this research and the committee's interest in child abuse and neglect was a large center grant application with the National Institutes of Health (P50 NICHD) that had a strong community-engaged component, which would not have been part of this vision had it not been formed in this collaborative interdisciplinary and community-engaged group. In a competitive process the project was scored and, while not selected for funding, the reviews were especially positive about the scope and quality of the community-engaged part of the proposal.

Chapter 9

Interdisciplinary Community-Engaged Research (ICER) for Health

Growing in Understanding and Effectiveness

Lina Svedin
University of Utah

Farrah Jacquez
University of Cincinnati

Chapter Context

This chapter takes stock of several lessons learned from the work presented across this volume. The teams that have been conducting interdisciplinary community-engaged research (ICER) for health show significant growth over time, as researchers, community partners, advocates, and policy leaders. While many teams faced challenges that seemed too daunting to tackle, and many had to return to the drawing board more than once, the collective experience evidenced in the preceding chapters tells us that it can be done. This chapter highlights key features of ICER in practice, and how you can make it work and contribute to the communities that make this type of research possible. We describe the primary themes that appeared across chapters to serve as a road map to navigate the challenges and reap the benefits of ICER.

Social Entrepreneurship for Change

Seeking to find not only innovative thinking for system-level change, social entrepreneurs also seek tangible ways to address the most pressing environmental, social, and cultural issues facing our communities today. Much like the Ashoka organization that the Birthing Project USA is modeled on, the kind of interdisciplinary community-engaged research for health that is covered in this volume identifies, supports, and promotes leading social entrepreneurship in the United States today. As social entrepreneurs, the teams presenting their work in this volume have persistently sought positive social change that will produce better health for children in America.

The Cincinnati team holds real-world change as a foundational value driving the work they do. By establishing early on that the research team in the project would involve the community as an equal research partner co-creating the research, not just transactional research, where the community is put under a microscope and studied, the team allayed CAKE members' early worries. The core value of CAKE, an equal partnership between community members and the research team, was key to the real-life change that was the project's primary outcome. The focus on action grew organically from naturally occurring policy changes happening in Cincinnati. A merged campaign run by the local Cincinnati Public School District (Cincinnati Preschool Promise, CPP) and a number of grassroots leaders got a petition passed in 2016 to offer universal preschool in Cincinnati. The successful advocacy and decision to grant access to quality preschools for kids was a historic win for the community and a testament to the collaborative effort. Along with the successful advocacy, the collaboration between the school district and the community also made it possible to hold those responsible for the distribution of funds accountable and making sure that the money reached those families in most need. The Cincinnati team saw this as "a unique opportunity to engage community leaders and neighborhood residents into evidence-based action to promote early childhood wellness" (chapter 3, p. 40).

The drive for social entrepreneurship in Indiana grew out of the issues at hand—the pervasiveness of incarceration and the negative impacts on children in Indiana. The community advocate learned of the fellowship opportunity and recruited researchers who could help policymakers see the link between mass incarceration and the state-level initiative to expand and advance pre-kindergarten. Through a snowball effect, the team came together with the diverse elements of expertise needed to impact a complex social problem. Because the members had no prior history of working together, they really became a team when they were selected to participate in the IRL program and received funding to do the proposed work.

For each team, a central element fueling the work was a need not only to make a real-world change but to understand how that change happens. The New York team (chapter 6) explicitly describes their process of diving deep into the theory of change that made their intervention work. Social entrepreneurship is change-oriented, and underlying and unvoiced assumptions sometimes clash with reality. Coming to terms with, and coming to an agreement on, the team's working theory of change was a cornerstone in designing and rolling out the intervention aimed to change the situation for poor mothers and pregnant women through Room to Grow, their intervention to support young mothers in New York City.

Research Teams under Construction

Any time you do anything with other people, it takes time to get it right. Investing time is required to build trust, to find ways to communicate effectively, and to align individual goals with a common effort. Research teams, it turns out, function the same way, no matter the individual participants' intelligence and expertise. Getting it right looked different for each team in this volume; however, all of them had to, at some point or another, get to know each other. The Arkansas team, like the Indiana team, had not worked together prior to the grant opportunity that made the community engaged research possible. Each of the Arkansas team members had a slightly different focus with regards to maternal health and well-being. These differences in focus and the fact that the members were thrown together in this venture the team felt worked as a positive and ended up being a strength of the team. They describe how their team's willingness to share their own personal experiences and biases allowed them to dig deeper into the biases, inequities, and social determinants of health of their local context and how these affect the health of their communities. As a team, they had to adjust the way they normally communicate, make efforts to include each other in a joint decision-making process, and come to agreements on what the team was going to do. Many times the collaboration process involved making mistakes, owning up to falling short, and assuming good intentions of other team members when the going got rough.

The Puerto Rico team had significant personnel changes that affected the ways team members were able to contribute to the project and required flexibility in research management plans. The community partner on their team changed positions within the organization and had much less capacity to develop the educational platform that was going to be disseminated throughout Puerto Rico's WIC program. One of the academic partners moved from Puerto Rico to a new institution in Florida, limiting her ability to contribute to work happening on the ground. The team worked together to identify new ways to manage funding so that the work could proceed as planned despite the changes in positions that are inevitable when successful people collaborate.

For the Utah team, the enthusiasm that they each brought to the shared effort was not enough to carry them through. Running headfirst into changing job responsibilities, different organizational demands and quirks along with three absolutely maxed-out schedules, the team relied heavily on their original team agreement to always assume good intentions. They also had to make this research happen in airports, over dinner in each other's homes, enlisting their children to babysit other team members' children, and trusting that the other partners were going to deliver on delegated tasks. They played to each members' strengths and tried to be as accommodating as possible knowing and understanding that they each had their own perspectives that brought something valuable. In other words, they trusted that their investment in the collaboration was worth it.

The Indiana team discovered the hard way that skipping team building early in the research process and not clarifying where each member was coming from can get quite painful. The team relied on each member being very experienced, well-connected, and having individually shown great leadership capabilities. The excitement they felt for the grant and fellowship had them glossing over the fact that neither of them really knew much about the other people on the team or their individual work. With the pressing deadline to submit the grant and fellowship application, the team members only managed some brief face-to-face meetings in pairs. They also had a couple of phone calls, but "the entire three-member team never met in person prior to the submission" (chapter 4, p. 63) of the application. As is often the case for funded research teams each member contributed to the proposal, addressed their specific area of expertise but in isolation and without coming together in a natural way to create a shared vision of the work at hand. This, however, meant that the team's "communication was disjointed from the beginning and over time this affected all aspects of the team progress" (chapter 4, p. 63). For this Indiana team, it got awkward enough that they had to stop and take stock of where they may have skipped a few steps in coming together as a research team. They found that they needed to go back and do some of that socioemotional labor in order to be able to keep moving forward with their project.

Finding and Creating Solutions

One of the real advantages of having an interdisciplinary research team with a community partner as a full research team member is the grounding and leverage it provides. The grounding of having a community partner continuously reflecting and bringing research ideas and questions into the context of community and practice secures relevance, feasibility, and usability. In the best of circumstances, it also allows for the cross-fertilization of community and practice needs with experiences and research results from other contexts and communities. The particularly ingenious combination of researchers from different disciplines working with community partners toward a common goal makes for a strong and dynamic set of experiences and knowledge. The interdisciplinary team can serve as a powerful source of strength that allows participants to push boundaries and think system-wide, a luxury seldom afforded to either practitioners or researchers in their day-to-day routine. This system-wide lens allows researchers and practitioners to identify what works.

For instance, several of the teams have, through the process of doing their community-engaged research, been able to use what works in local communities to address thorny and persistent social problems that negatively affect the health of young children. In Minnesota the interdisciplinary team has been trying to address inequity in birthing outcomes among the state's African American residents by partnering with Roots, an African American–owned and operated for-profit birthing clinic. It is a "best-practices clinic," with a home-like facility and working in a healthcare program designed on a wellness model of pregnancy and birth. It provides opportunities for many local women and their families to survive and thrive through pregnancy. The clinic and the work the group is doing could be replicated in other states that struggle with poor and inequitable birth outcomes. The potential for out-of-hospital births to reduce disparities experienced by African American women has not been adequately explored in the research literature. Partnering with the owner of the Roots clinic allowed the team to investigate the potential of out-of-hospital (deinstitutionalized) care by a healthcare provider that shares the cultural background of the mother to improve the birth experiences of African American women.

The Arkansas team has been trying to do research on maternal and infant health differently—in a way that contributes to maternal health in a community-centering and capacity-building way. The Arkansas team worked with the local affiliate of Birthing Project USA—a community-based and community-led mentoring program that provides social and emotional support prenatally and one year postnatal. The core of the program is building up capacity, building relationships, and assessing what works so that the community is left better off and with the tools in place to maintain the benefits for the long haul. The added value of the research team then is to support what is already being done, assess existing practices, suggest ways to strengthen and build on what is found to be effective, and help spread the word about this to other communities and geographic regions.

The Utah team has worked on translating ideas that have worked in other difficult circumstances to inform how organizations serving infants at risk of child abuse and neglect could possibly structure their work to collaborate better. The team purposely drew on research on crisis management collaboration, organizational psychology, and the idea of the family-centered medical home as a way to better support families who struggle socioeconomically. The team has been able to draw out lessons about what works and what does not in other states and put it up for consideration in Utah using a multi-method design. The team has also been able to innovate and pilot new collaborative practices to connect child welfare with the child because of the community partner, a state-run government agency, and its openness to evidence-based practices and a strong commitment to continuous improvement.

Defining Who "the Community" Is in ICER Projects

One of the first challenges the teams in this volume were faced with was defining who the community in their community-engaged research was. Who is the primary community partner? Who does that partner represent and who may be important to engage that may not be represented directly by the community partner in the team? Naming the community can be a delicate issue to navigate when communities are split along political, religious, or ethnic lines and the problems communities experience are not shared equally. Some teams were challenged by "missing" communities, where important stakeholders are physically removed from the conversations, as in the case with incarcerated parents, or hard to engage, as in the case with the caregivers of infants who have or have had child protective service (CPS) involvement. In spite of the challenges sometimes accompanying the question of who makes up the community we are interested in and want to engage, it is key to community-engaged research.

The primary community for the Puerto Rico team was the Puerto Rico WIC program (PR-WIC) as represented by the WIC coordinator Alexandra Reyes. The goal for the team's work was to find ways to promote healthy lifestyles among children participating in the PR-WIC program and to promote that families should embrace a culture of health to prevent early childhood obesity. However, as the WIC coordinator was reassigned to be a clinic supervisor, the team shifted focus to having whoever was functioning in the WIC leadership position as the community they were working with. Then, as Puerto Rico was hit by two catastrophic hurricanes a few months into the project, the team shifted focus again and came to consider the community that they worked with the WIC participants and the larger Puerto Rico population, and the team set out to support the WIC staff in their direct work to help people survive the effects of Hurricanes Irma and Maria. Designing and implementing self-care programs for WIC staff became part of the Puerto Rico team's work and doing what they could to support their community partner organization and its clinics; being engaged as community participants, the team was able to design ways to still get the data they were seeking— the process of getting there just ended up looking different than originally designed.

The Utah team, like many others, was trying to achieve a change in a target population through a community partner organization with good access to that population. The Utah team was initially quite intently focused on the goal of improving health outcomes for infants at risk of child abuse and neglect. A worthy and important focus to be sure, but the focus created a bit of a blind spot for the team. It was not until well into the research project that the team recognized that the primary community of their research effort was the CPS caseworkers at the front line of the child welfare agency. The team had been so focused on the goal—to improve health outcomes for at-risk infants—that they almost missed that a key target audience and stakeholder that needed to have input on (1) the goals of the research, (2) the processes of implementing pilots, and (3) reviewing the results, were the agency caseworkers themselves. While the team had correctly identified that CPS caseworkers were pivotal for initiating and making collaboration with child healthcare succeed, the team had to step back and recognize that even within this research project aimed to assess and support collaboration there were different communities that need to have input on the research process itself.

What both of these teams illustrate directly, and what is resonated in many other team's experience, is the need to be flexible in how community is viewed, delimited, and defined, even as a formal research project is well under way. The team's experience also reflects the fluidity of wanting to create change in one population or community, through a community partner organization. The community partner organization may or may not be part of the target population for the intervention or solution, which then posits questions about the appropriate level of engagement and participation of the population-based community in research design, implementation, and feedback. The answer to these questions is not always forthcoming and clear and seems to require considerable redress and reassessment at every stage of the research process.

Strengths-Based Approaches

Many teams described the critical need to focus on community assets and reject the traditional framing of "at-risk," problem-plagued, vulnerable populations. Rather than focusing on deficits and lacking resources in communities, all the teams featured took a strengths-based approach to the problem they were studying and trying to address. Looking for strengths in addressing community challenges and promoting health looked different in the specific projects. For instance, one of the Cincinnati team's core values is being asset-focused. They chose this core value because they knew the community had long experienced researchers coming in to diagnose community problems, without any investment in finding sustainable solutions An asset-based approach instead offered a way to identify and enhance household and community assets that already existed in these communities. The community partner organization in the Cincinnati team also had a great deal of experience already in using an asset-based approach. For example, the New Prospect Baptist Church, and its pastor, Damon Lynch, had already been using this approach to mobilize community members that came through his doors. The grassroots-driven nature of the Cincinnati early childhood health research project led to the promotion of resources and connecting parents to opportunities rather than focusing on researching the lack of resources.

What is evident from the narratives in the volume is also that the teams took a strengths-based approach to their own work and pragmatically drew on the strengths of each team member as the work ultimately demanded more of the team than they felt they could pull off. The strength of the Indiana team, they felt, was the task orientation—the ability to get stuff done both independently and together. The ability to complete tasks pretty efficiently allowed the team to progress even though the team's identity and ability to truly communicate was still seriously challenged. Thus, the team experienced success but in hindsight felt that they did so in a way that was harder than it needed to be. If the team had done the team-building exercises that were built into the fellowship curriculum attached to the grant, the team later said, they would have been so much better off. Time constraints and difficulty in scheduling time when the whole team could meet and spend time getting to know each other, develop relationships, and do exercises to get to know each other's work and collaborative style prevented the team from evolving from a task machine to a cohesive team. They stated, "In retrospect, it was clear that taking the time to get to know each team member and to discuss in detail our work and beliefs would create a stronger team and avoid problems down the road. The second lesson is 'No, really do… team building activities!'" (chapter 4, p. 67).

The Utah team developed a respect for the diverse expertise of the team early on, in part by walking in each other's shoes for periods of time, learning in the setting where the research partners worked, what it was like, and what that perspective brought to the interdisciplinary work of the team. The Utah team also quickly had to learn to manage and respect the team's different contexts and constraints as calendars filled to the rim and job positions and responsibilities kept shifting for the team members as they went through the research process.

Three teams in this volume have built their research on community-driven programs and services that have already demonstrated success. Through interdisciplinary community-academic partnerships, they were able to build on assets already existing in communities and expand the evidence base for their work. In Minnesota the interdisciplinary team has been trying to address inequity in birthing outcomes among the state's

African American residents by partnering with an African American–owned and operated for-profit birthing clinic, Roots. Roots is based on best practices, replicates a home environment, and is designed in line with a wellness model of pregnancy and birth. It provides opportunities for many local women and their families to survive and thrive through pregnancy. The clinic and the work the group is doing could be replicated in other states that struggle with poor and inequitable birth outcomes.

In New York City researchers at Columbia University paired with Room to Grow, a nonprofit serving families of children under three in order to conduct a randomized controlled trial to demonstrate the program's effectiveness and to document the aspects of Room to Grow's process that were driving impact (chapter 6). The program was already an asset to families of young children in the community; the interdisciplinary research partnership helped to provide evidence for outcomes and demystify the process, thereby capturing the magic that makes the intervention work.

The Importance of Relationships

The chapters and experiences in this volume communicate over and over again the importance of relationships. It is foundational to teamwork, even to forming a team and convincing others to join. The Utah ICER team came together because of the inherently and overtly collaborative nature of the Utah Child Welfare agency director at the time. His openness to building new relationships to improve the work the agency is doing made it possible for the associate director of the agency to become a fully participating research leader in this effort. By curious or cosmic alignment, one of the strongest findings from this team's research on interprofessional collaboration around infants at risk of maltreatment is the fundamental importance of relationships. The Utah team found that if personal relationships and connections do not exist, organizations do not collaborate or collaborate poorly. If a personal connection has been established between individuals in the organizations involved, however, collaboration can survive and thrive regardless of policy and regulatory environment.

The Cincinnati team started out very intentionally keeping the focus broad, primarily centered on improving early childhood wellness in the Roselawn and Carthage neighborhoods, so that the community's voice could shape the team's specific research questions. While the effort at inclusiveness was core to the team's approach, finding a target for intervention that cut across all stakeholders' priorities but was still a clear vision turned out to be very difficult. Trying to incorporate all priorities led to diffuse focus, which made it difficult to integrate into the larger context of early childhood advocacy efforts in Cincinnati. The Cincinnati team had decided to pay CAKE leaders for their participation in CAKE meetings, recognizing that everyone's time is valuable and in order to actively support community engagement. An important part of managing the relationship with CAKE members and building trust, the team eventually came to realize, included managing expectations. The team expected CAKE members to work outside of meetings as co-researchers, but they did not articulate those expectations specifically nor did they outline concrete goals with regards to the co-researcher role. As a consequence, the CAKE participants became unclear about what they were supposed to do outside of the meetings and how much they were expected to do, and they began to feel uncertain about the collaborative's accomplishments. Based on this experience the Cincinnati team reflected that it would have been better to create roles and expectations for each member collaboratively and then check back in each month to see the goal progress that each individual had made, rather than let unvoiced expectations undermine the developing relationship.

There were also several things that the Cincinnati team thought helped sustain the relationship between team members and the community as they were working together. Centering on the value of relationship-building as an integral part of the research process, providing resources for the community—such as providing food at meetings and funding, and making meetings as convenient and informative for everyone as possible—really helped maintain CAKE as a collaborative effort. Evaluation and self-reflection have also been a priority for the Cincinnati research team, including having an outside person conduct interviews with the community members in the collaborative to make sure the team was adhering to its espoused core values. The process of self-evaluation also identified areas where the team needed to be more effective in order to maintain the collaborative partnership. The evaluation showed that CAKE members were dissatisfied with the lack of tangible action, which the team tracked down to be rooted in the broad scope of the topic. The team came to recognize that improving early childhood well-being in these two communities was not specific enough to allow the team to make sufficient progress and generate tangible action that community members were looking for. In hindsight, the team recognized the need "to balance relationship-building and action and [be] more diligent about keeping track of progress on action steps and discussing them at each meeting" (chapter 3, p. 54).

Flexibility Needed

The stories relayed in this volume convey that one thing is certain in this type of work: uncertainty. Whatever thoughts and plans the teams had usually changed as the process of doing the work unfolded. This is not the clearly structured and neat work that many researchers learned as graduate students and may even have gotten used to working in labs or from the comfort of their office armchairs. This is messy, emotional, and rewarding work, where reality frequently interferes with the best-laid plans.

Several teams reflect on the need to change research plans, the focus of the whole research project, or methods by which answers and solutions to problems are sought. Team Puerto Rico jokingly argue that change has been the only constant over the course of their ICER project. The representative of the community partner organization, PR-WIC, played a very significant role in designing the intervention the team wanted to assess and was a named recipient of the grant that allowed the team to work together. Alexandra Reyes, the PR-WIC representative, was reassigned by PR-WIC to fill a different leadership function, which then did not allow her to continue in her ICER role. The lead research faculty member took a new job and moved states several months into the project. The grant was moved to a new organization, and one of the team members who remained in Puerto Rico had to take over the budget responsibility. The island was hit by two devastating hurricanes at the end of year one (of three) of the team's work. This changed every condition for the team's work, the community partner organization, and life on the island itself, down to not having electricity for several months. However, in spite of this, the team continued to work together, supporting each other, the community partner organization, and people in need. The Puerto Rico team's experience and take away from all this is that life happens—people will move to different institutions and organizations, policy changes, and this will require adaptation. In the midst of this, staying committed and being flexible is essential.

The Cincinnati team also managed to take away positive experiences from the need to be flexible in ICER work. For example, one of the best examples of the power of the Cincinnati's team's core value of shared decision-making involved the complete overhaul of proposed research activities. The team originally proposed a large household survey project, but the community members of the CAKE leadership team did not feel the huge investment required for that kind of individual-level research had a clear enough payoff for early childhood wellness in the Carthage and Roselawn neighborhoods. Together, the leadership team changed the research plan to focus survey efforts on providers in the neighborhoods instead.

At the same time, the Cincinnati group recognized that no process for decision-making in the CAKE collaborative had been established. Community CAKE members clearly had full membership and share in the decisions about where the research was going, but no actual process had been articulated for when or how decisions required a vote or a formal recognition that a decision had been made. The decision process that emerged in the CAKE meetings involved talking about important topics and issues as a full group and then to trust that those implementing the research were going to follow what the group seemed to agree on. The Cincinnati team thought that because one of the community CAKE members was a formal partner on the three-person research team there was enough trust in the group to proceed this informal way. The team also recognized, however, that if community members disagreed with things in the discussion they may not have brought that forward because there was no formal process for doing so or airing grievances outside of the group setting.

One thing that can be gleaned from the stories these teams relay is that you can be successful in this research as a research-community partnership if you stay committed to each other, to the partnership, and if you are flexible in the face of changing circumstances. If you expect change—not stability—in this work, the team can survive these curve-balls. The IRL-funded research teams were encouraged, as part of the fellowship, to do a series of team-building exercises at the outset of the research process. Many of the teams took the time to do this; however, many teams prioritized other tasks, found it difficult to set aside the time to do team-building, or felt very uncomfortable engaging in this type of personal and sometimes intimate sharing as part of a professional working group.

One of the team-building exercises that the IRL fellowship was encouraging the grant recipient teams to do was "a visual representation of team development based on a metaphor of a river" (chapter 4, p. 73). The Indiana team was reluctant to engage in this less task-oriented "art project" exercise, but after a while settled into creating a river mural with markers and paper. The process of creating the mural, with visual rep-resentations of the events, professional demands, and developments that had impacted the team so far, allowed the team to talk through the early challenges of their work together. It strengthened the team to collectively visualize and process those challenges, even down to the rocky founda-tion the team had built in terms of an identity and poor communication. The team-building art project helped the team acknowledge and own its stormy beginning, to recognize that the team was still okay and that the members were still committed to moving forward toward the goal they had established in the grant application: "We saw that our boat remained upright, and we remained committed to the cause" (chapter 4, p. 73). This gave the team hope that the completion of their research would be smoother because they had expressed some of their feelings, including the lack of team identity and their struggle to communicate effectively with each other.

The Minnesota team knew the importance of committing to each other and the work that they were going to do early on. At various points the team felt the pressure of keeping a for-profit birthing center afloat financially while delivering babies and doing community-engaged research at the same time. Team members' commitment to the vision of the research, their commitment to one another, and their commitment to the persons in the community who had been unmistakably impacted by structural and interpersonal racism while they were pregnant or giving birth were what kept the team together. Personal commitment to other persons and collectives can serve as a glue or extra energy source when the realities of doing research on very difficult and persistent issues, together as an academic-community partnership, get rough and start fraying the edges.

Bringing it Back

Somewhere in the middle of their collaborative research process, each of the teams featured in this volume had to start thinking about dissemination. How were they going to report what they found and to what audiences were they really speaking? Traditionally, researchers present their findings in publications—journal articles, book chapters, or full-length books. This is not, however, how most practitioners get new ideas. Policymakers spend, on average, ten minutes a day reading, and what they primarily read are not peer-reviewed journal articles but news articles. Academic publications, to researchers' surprise and dismay, are not experienced as very accessible or even relevant to practitioners and community organizers on the go.

There is also a history of community research being done without significant participation and input from community subjects themselves. Researchers study the community and its members in ways and for reasons that are not anchored in the community's own needs or desires. Not surprisingly, the results and findings from research done this way have also been kept in the realm that designed the study and not brought back to the community in any useful way. A common way for university research projects to be organized is that a principal investigator, a faculty member of a department or a research lab, designs the research and acquires funding for it. If it is funded, a team of graduate students or junior researchers then do the majority of the legwork in terms of the actual research—including recruiting participants and study subjects, and doing the actual measuring or testing that is at the center of the research project. The analysis and dissemination of findings rarely come back to the community where the research took place or to the research subjects themselves. Thus classic university studies tend to be marred by this transactional logic between researchers and the study subjects—the recognition and the credit of the advances of the research are heaped on the principal investigator. In most cases the community participants are left with only the hourly compensation for their participation, if that, and much less often with solutions to the challenges that prompted the researchers to sweep into their community.

Arkansas has seen this in maternal health and maternal mortality connected to pregnancy and birth. While many researchers who have wanted to make a difference with regard to maternal and infant mortality rates in the Mississippi Delta region have ties to the geographic area, many have frequently seen research in this area as a way to secure grant funding or to make a name for themselves. As a result, even the most idealistic research intentions frequently result in short interventions, where things are tested or done to women or to communities, largely without any substantive or lasting positive effect. The results may be disseminated in an academic journal, but the intervention and the research attention then go away, regardless of whether the research results were positive or negative. The community and the women are then left without having gained any tangible benefit at all as a result of the research they chose to support. As a consequence, residents are reluctant to participate in research or interventions because they perceive that researchers do not care to consider the real-world experiences of the people living in the community.

For all these reasons, disseminating findings and ideas outside of researchers' comfort zones, across traditional boundaries, and back to communities is an important and necessary component of interdisciplinary community-based research. The teams approached this differently and testify to various challenges and successes in this work. The Utah team learned the hard way that participating in conferences on child abuse and neglect for a policy scholar can be emotionally overwhelming and hard to process. This same team learned, however, that running workshops with minimal preparation and engaging in unstructured discussions with large audiences was something that stressed out the child abuse pediatrician and community partner. All three team members had to stretch to be able to communicate with the audiences that the other team members were very comfortable with, but they also had to learn to take cues from their partners about informal expectations and rules of engagement with audiences other than their own. Even the adjustment of language and use of terms was a constant adjustment as the team's research kept crossing disciplinary and organizational contexts.

The central goal for the Puerto Rico ICER team was to boost the dissemination of the WIC nutrition curriculum and to empower community member participants to develop healthy lifestyle choices. The team remained true to this goal throughout their project but were forced to be flexible in their dissemination plans when Hurricanes Irma and

Maria struck the island in September 2017 and left communities without power for several months. The team broadened their project's scope as it was evident that most people on the island were struggling with the post-hurricane living conditions. Service providers were facing WIC recipients' desperation and need while they were simultaneously trying to meet their own needs and those of their family members. They were victims of the disaster too. To boost morale and do what they could as true collaborating partners, the Puerto Rico research team decided to facilitate a self-care workshop for the staff of the PR-WIC nutrition program. The team also helped develop the dissemination posters used to advance the nutritional curriculum, which were used to engage clinics throughout Puerto Rico. The Puerto Rico team's ability to be flexible and responsive to community needs was enhanced by the interdisciplinary diversity of their team and their strong partnership with the larger WIC program on the island.

Choosing the Road Less Traveled: The Future of ICER for Health

The history of research in communities to fix problems identified by people on the outside, those who do not live the lives of those in the community, is long and marred by problems and distrust. There has been a lot of inappropriate and harmful research done to people and communities; experiences that have deepened suffering and left communities without resources to move forward. What the teams in this volume have tried to do is different. They have done the messy, emotionally invested work of trying to address hard and persistent challenges to early childhood health and well-being. Not with children or communities as test subjects but with community organizations as full research partners, invested in the design of the research, the analysis of information about their community, and in getting what the research yielded back to the community in which they live.

The work that has been presented in this volume takes on astonishingly complex and persistent challenges to the health of young children. There is inherent value to improving health—building a culture of health—across the United States, and we support that. However, these researchers do work to improve the lives of children, because early childhood health and well-being represents a unique leveraging point for future health and a population-wide shift in how we think about and integrate health as a cultural value. Early childhood adversity has a direct link to long-term health problems that then impact future children and their families. If we can be socially entrepreneurial, and innovate, trust, and collaborate around at-risk children, we have a shot at making a difference on downstream health outcomes. By designing interventions, programs, and networks to promote early childhood well-being *with* communities, we can make the change sustainable.

What the teams in this volume are doing is action research in many ways, with much shorter timelines than academic researchers frequently operate under, but much longer timelines than community organizers typically live with. It has required team-building, being open and honest about what can and cannot be done, what team members are familiar with, and what they have no idea how to do. It involves not just the more removed study of something but trying to have an impact—whether that is through community building, bringing awareness and connecting community members to resources, talking to policymakers, writing op-ed pieces, or having a voice in settings that the team members normally do not enter. For community partners, allowing someone from the outside who does not know as much about the work you do come in and look at *how* you do something and how it might be improved or sustained is both valuable and difficult. It requires a lot of trust for a partner to connect their community to people who, even with good intentions, may not have the experience required to reach that community or understand the complexity of what members face every day. All of these things require stretching, trusting, and growing—things that are frequently forgotten or overlooked when partners are operating from their professional point of view.

Interdisciplinary community-engaged research is not for the faint of heart, but it is absolutely worth it. A necessary step to making interdisciplinary community-engaged research easier, more accepted in academia, and more useful to communities and practitioners, we offer this book as a road map. The team's experiences, projects, implementation plans, and revised plans offer shortcuts, gaps to be mindful of, and ways out of the challenges that are bound to arise if you want to start this kind of work. Our hope is that this will be a useful stepping stone for many students, change leaders, community organizers, policymakers, and researchers who want to improve life, culture, and health in the United States. We look forward to sharing this path with you as you join us on the frontlines of interdisciplinary community-engaged research for health.

Bios

Editor Bios

Farrah Jacquez, PhD is a professor and Assistant Head of the Department of Psychology at the University of Cincinnati. Her work focuses on community-engaged approaches to health equity and broadening participation in science and research. Dr. Jacquez works with community members as partners in research to develop evidence-based, contextually appropriate intervention programs and push for tangible systems level change to promote wellness. She currently has several funded projects that use participatory research methods to include community stakeholders in research processes. She is the PI of an NIH-funded Science Education Partnership Award (SEPA) that engages adolescents in rural Appalachia and urban Cincinnati in community-based participatory research on drug abuse and addiction in local communities. She also serves as the co-PI of a Community Conversations grant from the Corporation for National and Community Service that partners with refugees as co-researchers to improve civic engagement of refugee populations in Cincinnati. Dr. Jacquez was part of the first cohort of the Interdisciplinary Research Leaders fellowship with the Robert Wood Johnson Foundation and currently serves on the Board of Directors for Community-Campus Partnerships for Health (CCPH). She is Co-Director of Community Engagement for the Center for Clinical and Translational Science and Training (CCTST), an organization funded by the Clinical and Translational Science Award (CTSA) by the NIH.

Lina Svedin, PhD is an associate professor in the Department of Political Science at the University of Utah. Lina is Swedish by origin and has worked both as an area specialist for the Swedish national government, and as a research leader and training director at the Swedish National Center for Crisis Research and Training. A majority of her research has focused on governance challenges in crisis conditions including ethics and accountability in the distribution and management of societal risk. Much of her current research focuses on taboo topics in public policy, including homelessness, suicide, child sexual abuse and economic inequality, and the impact of policy on marginalized populations. Dr. Svedin teaches administrative theory, policy analysis, program evaluation, ethics for public administrators, as well as governance and the economy in the Master of Public Policy and the Master of Public Administration programs. Dr. Svedin was part of the first cohort of the Interdisciplinary Research Leaders fellowship with the Robert Wood Johnson Foundation and is currently on an Intergovernmental Personnel Act assignment to the School of Advanced Air and Space Studies at Air University, Maxwell AFB. Prior to this assignment, she was the Director of Public Affairs Programs, College of Social and Behavioral Science at the University of Utah.

Contributor Bios

Chapter 2: Enhancing the Arkansas Birthing Project through Technology

Zenobia Harris, DNP, RN is the Executive Director of the Arkansas Birthing Project and has been a public health practitioner/administrator for 35 years. Her work involves empowering community members to participate in meaningful ways to encourage greater civic engagement in the change process.

Sarah Rhoads, PhD, DNP, WHNP-BC is a professor at the University of Tennessee Health Science Center. Her work examines ways to improve access to care to rural and underserved areas using technology while remaining true to the community.

Hari Eswaran, PhD is a professor and Director of Research at the Institute of Digital Health and Innovation, University of Arkansas for Medical Sciences, and has worked in the area of maternal and fetal monitoring for the last 25 years. His work focuses on the areas of research, design, and innovation in healthcare technology, and data analytics.

Chapter 3: A Place-Based Approach to Early Childhood Wellness in Cincinnati: Communities Acting for Kids Empowerment (CAKE)

Michael Topmiller, PhD is a Health GIS Research Specialist at Health-Landscape, a division of the American Academy of Family Physicians, and a recent graduate of the Robert Wood Johnson Foundation's Interdisciplinary Research Leaders fellowship program. Michael's areas of expertise include population health, community-based participatory research (CBPR), and geospatial analysis.

Farah Jacquez (see above bio)

Jamie-Lee Morris is an aspiring writer and spoken word artist. The wealth of insight Jamie-Lee has gained from working directly with the community has helped shape who she is as a writer. Jamie-Lee is currently the Manager of Education and Outreach at Elementz Hip Hop Youth Center. Within Elementz, she functions as the lead organizer of the City-wide Poetry slam "Louder Than a Bomb Cincy" and the southwestern regional "Poetry Out Loud" contest.

Chapter 4: Finding Our Way as a Cross-Systems Team: Lessons Learned from an Interdisciplinary Research Team

Karen Ruprecht is a Managing Director, Early Childhood Systems for the State Child Care Capacity Building Center. Her field and scholarly work includes training and coaching early childhood professionals and researching quality initiatives that serve children and families with a focus on how research can inform policy and practice.

Angela Tomlin is a professor of Clinical Pediatrics at Indiana University School of Medicine. Her clinical and scholarly work includes training a wide range of professionals and researching reflective supervision and consultation to build and support a workforce prepared to serve high need families with young children.

Shoshanna Spector is Executive Director of Faith in Indiana. Through grassroots organizing, narrative development, and large-scale voter engagement efforts, Faith in Indiana has built the power to win policies to advance racial and economic justice. A Robert Wood Johnson Culture of Health alumni, Ms. Spector draws on 20+ years' experience in community organizing and social change.

Chapter 5: Improving Racial Equity in Birth Outcomes: A Community-Based, Culturally Centered Approach

Katy B. Kozhimannil, PhD, MPA is Associate Professor at the University of Minnesota School of Public Health. Her research informs clinical and policy strategies to advance racial, gender, and geographic equity. Dr. Kozhimannil collaborates with stakeholders in making policy change to facilitate improved health and well-being, starting at birth.

Rachel R. Hardeman, PhD, MPH is a reproductive health equity researcher whose program of research applies the tools of population health science and health services research to elucidate a critical and complex determinant of health inequity—racism. Her work has elicited critical evidence on the topics of culturally-centered care, police brutality, and structural racism as a fundamental cause of health inequities.

Rebecca Polston, CPM, LM is the owner and director of Roots Community Birth Center. She has a passion for building the Roots community and creating a safe space for all birthing families. She has been in practice for 6 years. She loves providing nurturing grounding care. She and her husband have 3 children, 2 of whom were born at home. She loves horses, her dog and reading.

Chapter 6: Creating Transformational Nonprofit/University Partnerships in Public Health: Lessons Derived from Collaboration between Room to Grow and Columbia University

Allyson Crawford is the CEO of Room to Grow. She has spent the last 20 years leading community organizations, classrooms, teams, and individuals to reach their highest possible potential. Her expertise includes human capital development, program design and evaluation, social change-centered strategy, partnership building, systems development, and social justice entrepreneurship.

Bethany Brichta is the National External Relations Director at Room to Grow, holding several roles at the organization since joining the team in 2014. A graduate of the University of Michigan, Bethany has spent the last 10 years in the nonprofit sector, with a focus on community engagement and fundraising.

Ruby L. Engel is a Research Analyst at the CPRC and CPSP at Columbia University. Engel is currently the Lead Research Coordinator for the Columbia Study of Mothers and Babies. She is particularly interested in the research areas of Reproductive Health and Maternal and Infant Wellness.

Joanna Groccia is the Senior Coordinator of Innovation and Strategy at Room to Grow. Joanna joined Room to Grow in 2014 and currently oversees program data and evaluation across the organization and helps to drive the implementation of Room to Grow's strategic growth plan.

Anna E. Holt, Room to Grow

Tonya Pavlenko, Center on Poverty and Social Policy, Columbia University School of Social Work

Karen Sanchez is an alumna and former research assistant for Columbia University. Her primary role was interviewing and collecting data for Spanish-speaking participants in the study. She currently works as a teaching associate for the Ross School.

Christopher Wimer is Senior Research Scientist and co-Director of the Center on Poverty and Social Policy at Columbia University. His work focuses on the measurement of poverty and disadvantage and the role of social policies and programs in promoting wellbeing among low-income individuals and families.

Chapter 7: Building Strong Partnerships with the Puerto Rico WIC Program for Promoting Healthy Lifestyles in Early Childhood and a Long-Lasting Culture of Health

Maribel Campos, MD is a pediatrician with Subspecialty in Neonatal and Perinatal Medicine and Diplomate in Obesity Medicine. As Professor of the University of Puerto Rico, her work focuses on the effects of early life exposures on health across the lifespan, and community action projects fostering a culture of health through science education and mindfulness strategies.

Cristina Palacios, PhD, MSC, is an associate professor in the Department of Dietetics & Nutrition at Florida International University. Her research focuses on the influence of diet on obesity and weight gain in infants, children, adolescents, and pregnant women. She is a consultant for the World Health Organization.

Alexandra Reyes, MEd, RDN is a Registered Dietitian Nutritionist in the WIC Program of Puerto Rico. She is an expert in nutrition education, breastfeeding, pregnancy and child nutrition and infant feeding practices.

Chapter 8: In Search of Child Welfare and Child Health Collaboration

Lina Svedin (see above bio)

Tonya Myrup, MSW, is the deputy director of the Division of Child and Family Services, Salt Lake City, Utah.

Kristine Campbell, MD MS is a general pediatrician, child abuse pediatrician, researcher and advocate in the Department of Pediatrics at the University of Utah. Her interest in social determinants of health grew from experiences in medical school (Johns Hopkins, 1991–1996), residency (University of Washington, 1996–1999), and practice on the Navajo reservation (1999–2004).

Index

f in index refers to footnote

A
action research, 6
Adverse Childhood Experiences (ACEs), 12
African American community
    low birth weight of infants, *vs.* white, 90
    mortality rate of infants, *vs.* white, 87
    newspaper, 98
    obesity rate of, 151
    out-of-hospital birth options, 86, 199
    population of Carthage and Roselawn,
        41
    unethical research practiced on, 85
    use of hospitals for childbirth, 85–86
    use of midwives in, 85–86
    see also Arkansas Birthing Project;
        Roots Community Birth Center
aging, 90
agricultural capacity, 49
alcohol abuse, 169
American Indian infants, 87
American Journal of Health, Ethnicity and Disease, 8
American Journal of Managed Care
    blog series, 84, 101
    website, 96
AmeriCorps, 49
android tablets, 31
Arkansas Birthing Project
    as affiliate of Birthing Project USA, 22,
        23, 25–28, 32–33, 199
    changes implemented, 199–200
    dissemination of research, 32–33,
        212–13
    funding for, 24

    research challenges and successes, 30–32
    research methods for, 30
    research team evaluation, 196
    team members and collaboration, 21–25
    use of technology in, 14, 21–22, 24,
        28–31, 33
Ashoka organization, 28, 198
asset-focused approach and values, 36, 37,
        39, 41, 44–47, 49, 52, 203
Association of Women's Health
        Obstetrical and Neonatal Nurses, 33
"As We Mourn Infant Death, Let's Take
        Care of Moms," (blog post), 101
attorneys, 173, 177, 180

B
baby goods and gear, 114, 115, 119
Balzacs, Carolina, 8–9
Battered Child Syndrome, 169
birth control, 29
birth inequity. *see* Roots Community Birth
    Center
birthing centers. *see* Roots Community
    Birth Center
Birthing Project USA (BPUSA)
    and Arkansas Birthing Project, 22, 23,
        25–28, 32–33, 199
    and dissemination of research
        collaboration, 32–33
    international projects, 27–28
    modeled on Ashoka organization, 28,
        194
    program model, 26–28
    web site, 27

"black box" of effects, 133

Black Lives Matter, 88

Black Maternal Health Week, 99

blogs, 84, 96, 101

BMI (body mass index), 150–51

books and book chapters, 211

Boston, 113, 115

Boston Opportunity Agenda's Birth
    Through Eight Collective, 143

breastfeeding, 29, 148, 151, 153

Bronx, New York, 137

Brooklyn, New York, 138

Brooks-Gunn, Jeanne, 117, 120, 128–30

Brownsville, New York, 138

Bunches (mentoring program), 26, 29–30

C

CAB. see community advisory board

CAKE. see Communities Acting for Kids
    Empowerment

California State Department of Health, 25

Campbell, Kristine, 167, 171, 182, 184,
    187–92

Campos, Maribel, 147, 154, 157, 160

Canino, Jeanette, 162

Carthage, Ohio
    asset-mapping project with
        AmeriCorps, 49
    GLA's in, 47
    Hispanic population in, 41, 42, 47
    monthly lunch meetings held at, 46
    reason for selection in CAKE research,
        37, 40–42, 51, 54, 206, 209
    selection of community members from,
        42
    sustainability of CAKE in, 49

Carthage Christian Church, 41, 46

cash assistance, 126

cellular data, 31

center-based model, 135

centering at the margins, 84

child health
    impact of mass incarceration upon,
        14–15, 62
    and obesity, 12, 148–55, 159, 161, 163
    as target area for IRL program, 12–13
    see also specific research projects

Child Protective Services (CPS). see Utah
    child welfare and child health
    collaboration research

churches
    and Arkansas Birthing Project, 27
    CAKE meetings held at, 46
    as community assets, 45
    group-level assessments held at, 47
    and parental incarceration, 57
    and youth music programs, 50
    see also specific churches

Cincinnati, Ohio. see Communities Acting
    for Kids Empowerment

Cincinnati College Conservatory of Music,
    50

Cincinnati Preschool Promise (CPP), 40,
    44, 49, 194

Cincinnati Public School District, 194

clearinghouses, 132

Clinical and Translational Science, 8

coaching support to parents, 114–15, 121

Collaborations: A Journal of Community-
    Based Research and Practice, 8

college and preschool attendance, 12

Columbia Study of Mothers and Babies, 15

Columbia University. School of Social
    Work
    Center on Poverty and Social Policy, 120
    collaboration with Room to Grow, 15,
        111–12, 113–20, 123–27, 133, 135,
        139, 143, 205

Columbia University. Teachers College,
    117, 120

Commission to Eliminate Child Abuse
    and Neglect Fatalities (2016), 172
communication differences, 70–72, 79
Communities Acting for Kids
    Empowerment (CAKE)
    as CAB-co-researcher hybrid model, 36,
        37–40, 42–44, 49–51
    and community organization in, 14
    core values, 43, 44–49, 52, 53, 194, 203
    funding for, 37, 39, 49–50, 54
    importance of collaboration in, 206–7
    maintenance stage of, 36, 39, 49–50,
        53–54
    selection of community members for, 42
    self-evaluation and plans for sustain-
        ability, 49–50, 209
    social entrepreneurship for change in,
        194–95
    team members, 35
    see also Carthage, Ohio; Roselawn, Ohio
community
    defined, for Utah child welfare
        research, 177, 201–2
    defined for ICER projects, 200–202
community advisory board (CAB)
    as co-researcher hybrid model, 42–44,
        51–54
    core values and CAKE operations, 43,
        44–49, 52, 53, 194, 203
    maintenance processes for, 36, 39,
        49–50, 53–54
    project lessons learned, 51–54
    replication of, 50–51
    three domains of, 38–39
community-based participatory research
    (CBPR)
    analysis of, 10
    definitions and practice, 5–8
    improving ways of conducting, 3–5
    journals for, 8

primary goals, 6
for Puerto Rico WIC research, 160–61
reasons for, 8–11
resources for collaboration, 16–18
in Room to Grow research, 138
terminology used by public health and
    academic medicine, 6
Community-Campus Partnerships for
    Health, 8
community partners as co-researchers, 36,
    37
confidentiality, 180
control group
    for Room to Grow, 118–19, 133, 138,
        139–40
    for Utah child welfare research, 169
core values
    of CAKE research, 43, 44–49, 52, 53,
        194, 203
    of Room to Grow and Columbia
        University, 143
CPP. see Cincinnati Preschool Promise
CPS (Child Protective Services). see Utah
    child welfare and child health
    collaboration research
"creaming myth," 124, 126
CTSA program (NIH Clinical and
    Translational Science Award), 7
Cuba, 28
curriculum
    fellowship, 204
    parenting, 141
    for Room to Grow, 121, 135
    standardized nutritional education for
        WIC program, 148, 149–50

D
databases
    HOMEVEE, 132
    for Room to Grow research, 122, 124, 125

data collection
    for Arkansas Birthing Project, 36
    for CAKE research, 38
    and collaborating with community
        members, 9
    for Indiana mass incarceration research,
        59, 76
    for Room to Grow research, 118,
        121–22, 133, 134–40
    for Roots Community Birth Center
        research, 99
DCFS. see Utah Division of Child and
    Family Services
decision making
    in Arkansas Birthing Project, 196
    in CAKE research, 36, 38–40, 43–45,
        47–50, 52–53, 209
    in community-academic partnerships, 6
    in Indiana mass incarceration research,
        69
    in Roots Community Birth Center
        research, 105
    in Utah child welfare research, 173
Delibertis, Jodi, 86
diabetes, 90
diversity
    among midwives, 86
    of team members, 66, 214
domestic violence shelters, 135
doulas
    community-based project, 94
    training for at Roots Community Birth
        Center, 93
dreaming ceremony, 27
drug abuse, 169

E
Early Childhood Collaborative, 143
early childhood education (ECE), 141
educators, 6, 177, 178

electricity, 158, 163, 208
electronic forms, 122, 125
electronic media, 157. see also specific media
emails
    for CAKE research, 47, 53
    in Indiana mass incarceration research,
        71, 72, 75
    in Puerto Rico WIC research, 157
    in Room to Grow research, 112, 125, 139
    in Roots Community Birth Center
        research, 95
    in Utah child welfare study, 181
employment, full-time, 12
Eswaran, Hari, 21–22, 24, 28, 32–33

F
Facebook, 139
Faith in Indiana, 57
family/friend contact, 139
family violence and dysfunction, 169
fatalities. see Utah child welfare and child
        health collaboration research
faxes, 124, 125
fellowship
    in Arkansas Birthing Project, 31
    in CAKE research, 39
    for Indiana mass incarceration research,
        62–68, 70, 75, 78, 195, 197, 203–4
    in Room to Grow research, 120
    and team-building exercises, 204, 210
field guide, 61
Florida International University, 154,
        156–57
focus group, 79
food
    for caregivers' meeting, 188–89
    insecurity, 137, 142, 157
food stamps, 126
formation of CABs, 38, 43, 51–52
Foster, Jennifer, 86

foster care placement, 170
freestanding birth centers, 86, 91
Frontiers in Innovation, 130
funding
    for child welfare, 174
    for federal home visiting programs, 131,
        132
    nonprofits' evaluation and, 132
    see also specific projects

G
*Gateways: International Journal of
    Community Research and Engagement,*
    8
Geronimus, Arline, 89–90
GLAs. *see* group-level assessments
granny midwives, 85
grant proposals
    community-engaged research as
        requirement in, 7
    with the National institutes of Health,
        192
    see also specific funding sources
group-level assessments (GLAs), 41–42,
    47–48

H
Hall-Trujillo, Kathryn, 25, 28
Hardeman, Rachel, 83, 98–99, 101, 103
Harris, Zenobia, 21, 23, 24–25, 28, 32–33
Harvard Center for the Developing Child,
    130
healthcare providers, 22, 161, 163, 168, 172,
    177
health inequity, 90, 91
Health Promotion Practice, 8
Hispanics
    and CAKE research, 41, 42, 47, 51
    see also Puerto Rico WIC research

HOMEVEE. *see* United States Health and
    Human Services Home Visiting
    Evidence of Effectiveness
home visiting programs, 131, 132
hospitals
    African American *vs.* white women's
        use of, for childbirth, 85–86
    in Arkansas Birthing Project, 27
    in Roots Community Birth Center, 84,
        85–86, 92
housing, 29, 90, 115
    public, 37, 126, 136
    unstable, 135, 137, 138, 142
"How Health Plans Can Support Moms"
    (blog post), 101
Hurricane Irma, 15–16, 149, 157–58, 163,
    201, 208, 213–14
Hurricane Maria, 15–16, 149, 157–58, 163,
    201, 208, 213–14
hybrid program model
    CAKE and CAB co-researcher model,
        36–40, 42–43, 50–51
    Room to Grow as, 140
hypertension, 90

I
ICER. *see* Interdisciplinary Community-
    Engaged Research
illegal substance use, 134
Indiana mass incarceration research
    conceptualization phase, 68–73
    and drive for social entrepreneurship
        in, 195
    forming the interdisciplinary team,
        62–64
    funding for, 62
    goals and methods, 57–58
    identifying a model for, 61–62
    impact of pre-k education, 14–15
    implementation phase, 73–77

Indiana mass incarceration research *(cont.)*
  incarcerated parents, 57–58, 69, 74, 79,
      185, 200
  role of interdisciplinary team for, 59–61
  team building, 65–66, 73, 197–98, 204,
      210
  team development phase, 64–68
  team members, 197–98
  time pressure, 67
  translation phase, 78–81
infants
  abuse and neglect of, 16
  and community stakeholders around
      at-risk, 176–83
  low birth weight, of African American
      infants *vs.* white, 90
  mortality and morbidity rates, 32, 87,
      93, 101, 103, 212
  and obesity, 12, 148–55, 159, 161, 163
insider researcher models, 38
Institute for Education Science's What
      Works, 132
Institute for Perinatal Quality
      Improvement initiative, 32
Institutional Review Board (IRB), 74, 79,
      127, 139, 186
Interdisciplinary Community-Engaged
      Research (ICER)
  defining "community" in projects,
      200–202
  dissemination of research, 211–14
  evaluation of research teams, 196–98
  finding and creating solution for,
      198–200
  flexibility needed in, 207–11
  future of, 214–16
  importance of relationships in, 80,
      205–7
  key features of, 193
  road maps for, 16–18

social entrepreneurship for change in,
      194–95
  strengths-based approaches to, 203–5
  see also fellowship
Interdisciplinary Research Leaders (IRL)
      program. Robert Woods Johnson
      Foundation
  and Arkansas Birthing Project, 24
  and CAKE research, 37, 39, 50, 54
  composition of IRL teams, 1–2
  early childhood health as target area,
      12–13
  and Indiana mass incarceration
      research, 62
  and Puerto Rico WIC research, 150,
      154, 157, 160
  requirements of, 2
  team building exercises for, 210–11
  Utah child welfare and child health
      collaboration research, 167, 172,
      183–91
interdisciplinary teams
  differences among members, 59–61
  identifying a model for, 61–62
internet, 153, 158
interviews
  with incarcerated parents, 185
  phone, 186
  for Puerto Rico WIC research, 155,
      196–97
  for Room to Grow research, 132–33, 136
iPads, 31
iPhones, 138
IRB. *see* Institutional Review Board
IRL. *see* Interdisciplinary Research
      Leaders program. Robert Woods
      Johnson Foundation
Irving, Shalon, 99
Irving, Soleil, 99
"ivory-tower" education research, 12

J
Jacquez, Farrah, 35, 41
jails. *see* Indiana mass incarceration
        research
journal articles, 211
Journal of Cancer Education, 8
*Journal of Healthcare for the Poor and
        Underserved,* 8
Journal of Midwifery & Women's Health, 86
Journal of Urban Health, 8
judges, 177

K
Karbeah, J'Mag, 83
Kozhimannil, Katy, 83, 94, 98–99, 101, 103

L
language
        barriers in shelter system, 136
        differences among team members, 188
        used on surveys, 134
Latinos. *see* Hispanics
law enforcement officers, 173, 177
lawsuits, 178f
lay researchers, 38
legislation
        pending in Utah, 190
        to reduce child abuse and neglect,
                174–75
        to support maternal mortality review,
                101
literature
        in CAKE research, 37–38
        collaboration on scientific, 9
        in community-engaged research, 9–11
        effect of disparate researchers'
                vocabulary on, 10
        on out-of-hospital births, 199
        in Room to Grow research, 130
        in Roots Community Birth Center
                research, 90

Little Sisters (Birthing Project mentees),
        26–27, 29–30, 31–32
"Lost Mothers" (documentary), 99
lunches
        for CAKE leadership teams, 46
        free and reduced, 41
        for Utah research team and CPS
                caseworkers, 182
Lynch, Damon, 203

M
Malawi, 28
Martin, Nina, 99
mass incarceration. *see* Indiana mass
        incarceration research
Maternal, Infant and Early Childhood
        Home Visiting (MIECHV), 131
maternal mortality, 22, 32, 98–99, 101, 103,
        212–13
        see also Arkansas Birthing Project
media coverage, 98–99
Medicaid, 93, 96
medical providers, 173
mental health in adults, 12
mentorship
        Arkansas Birthing Project, 26–27,
                29–30, 31–32
        Rose Community Birth Center, 102–3
metrics
        anthropometrics in Puerto Rico WIC
                research, 159
        in Room to Grow research, 116, 121, 143
midwives
        in African American community, 85, 86
        media recruitment for, 98
        mentoring for, 102–3
        training at Roots Community Birth
                Center, 93
        white women's use of, 86
MIECHV. *see* Maternal, Infant and Early
        Childhood Home Visiting

Minnesota
    birthing center in Minneapolis, 15
    childbirth care and outcomes in, 94–97
    legislation on prenatal care, 101
    media coverage in, 98
    midwives of color in, 102
Minnesota Birth Workers of Color, 94
Minnesota Black Chamber of Commerce,
    93
Minnesota Department of Health (MDH),
    87, 88
Minnesota Spokesman-Recorder, 98
Mississippi Delta Region, 22–23, 212
models of care
    Birthing Project, 28
    CAB/CAKE co-researcher model,
        36–44, 50–51
    in Indiana mass incarceration research,
        61–62, 78
    Puerto Rico WIC research, 149, 155,
        160, 161
    Room to Grow, 15, 112, 114–23, 126–27,
        129, 135–36, 140–41, 143
    Roots Community Birth Center, 15, 28,
        84–86, 89–94, 96, 106, 199, 205
    and social entrepreneurship, 194
    traditional, 184
Morello-Frosch, Rachel, 8–9
Morris, Jamie-Lee, 35, 41, 46
mortality rates
    infant, 32, 87, 93, 101, 103, 212
    maternal, 22, 32, 98–99, 101, 103,
        212–13
Myrup, Tonya, 167–68, 171, 176–77,
    181–86, 189–91

N
National Institutes of Health
    on benefits of collaboration, 6–7
    Clinical and Translational Science
        Award (CTSA), 7

and community involvement for
        funding, 50
    and Puerto Rico WIC research, 157
    and Utah child welfare research, 192
National Office of Families with Young
        Children, 118
National Ray Helfer Society, 190
National WIC Association, 158
Neighborhood Development Center, 93
New Prospect Baptist Church, 41, 46, 203
newsletters, 181
New York City, 113, 115, 125–26, 133, 135,
        143, 205
New York City Poverty Tracker, 137
Northside Economic Opportunity
        Network, 93
notary signature, 180
"Nothing Protects Black Women from
        Dying in Pregnancy and Childbirth,"
        99
nutrition education
    as reason for participating in WIC
        program, 153
    in Roots Community Birth Center, 106
    WIC as community-based nutritional
        program, 152
    see also Puerto Rico WIC research

O
obesity, adult, 147
obesity, childhood
    in Puerto Rico, 148, 149–52, 154, 155,
        159, 161, 163, 201
    rates in United States, 12, 150–51
operation of CABs
    and CAKE research, 52–53
    as one of best processes of, 37, 38–39
"Our Maternity Care System Is Broken:
        Here's How We Can Fix It." (blog
        post), 101
out-of-hospital births, 86, 199

P

Palacios, Christina, 147–48, 154, 156–57, 160

parents
accused of abuse and neglect, 173
coaching support to, 114–15, 121
and confidentiality, 180
incarcerated, 57–58, 69, 74, 79, 185, 200
one-on-one coaching for, 114, 121
perception of CPS, 169
survey results of satisfaction, 129

participatory action research, 6

pass-the buck exercises, 47–48

Pavlenko, Tonya, 142

payment policies for childbirth, 96, 97, 101, 106

PCORI (Patient-Centered Research Institute), 7–8

Peabody Award, 99

pediatricians, 16, 147, 167, 171, 190, 213

peer researchers, 38

phones, 139, 186

PI. *see* principal investigator

policymakers, 211

Polston, Rebecca, 83, 93, 94, 101, 104

postpartum period, 84, 92

prenatal care
as important determinant of maternal-infant outcomes, 88, 90
inadequate, 90
Little Sister-Sister Friend mentoring for, 26–27
racial disparities in, 101
single-payment reimbursement for, 106
technology for monitoring, 21

preschools and preschoolers
in Cincinnati, 14, 40
effect of parental incarceration upon, 57–58, 62
effect upon future college attendance, 12

effect upon future full-time employment, 12
importance of high-quality, 12
taxes for, 14

Preventing Maternal Deaths Act, 101

principal investigator (PI), 115

Progress in Community Health Partnerships, 8

ProPublica, 99

public assistance, 126

public housing, 37, 126, 136

Puerto Rico WIC research
and childhood obesity, 148, 149–52, 154, 155, 159, 161, 163, 201
dissemination of research, 213–14
effect of hurricanes upon, 15–16, 149, 157–58, 163, 201–208, 213–14
evaluation of research, 159–63, 207
evaluation of research team, 196–97
improving and continuing partnership, 155–58
key elements and challenges of program, 148–49, 152–54
phases of project, 154–55
primary community for, 201
research team members, 147
surveys for, 153, 155, 160

Q

Queens, New York, 137

R

racism
effect of weathering and birth equity, 89–91, 103
and effect upon birth outcomes, 94–97
media portrayals of, 100
structural, 15, 85, 88, 93, 97, 99, 107, 211

randomized control trials (RCT)
electronic referral forms, 125
for Room to Grow research, 115–19, 133

RCT. *see* randomized control trials

real-world change, 44, 45–46

recreation centers, 48

referrals
    to community resources, 114–15, 119,
        124, 125
    electronic versions, 125
    to partners, 139
    for suspected child abuse or neglect,
        173

rental assistance, 126

Reyes, Alexandra, 148, 154, 155–56, 159,
    160, 201, 208

Rhoads, Sarah, 21, 23–25, 29, 32

river mural team-building exercise, 210

Robert Wood Johnson Foundation
        program. Interdisciplinary Research
        Leaders (IRL)
    composition of IRL teams, 1–2
    Culture of Health conference, 142
    emphasis on early childhood health,
        12–13
    funding for Arkansas Birthing Project,
        24
    funding for CAKE research, 37, 39,
        49–50, 54
    funding for Indiana mass incarceration
        research, 62
    funding for Puerto Rico WIC research,
        150, 154, 157, 160
    funding for Room to Grow, 120, 127
    funding for Utah child welfare and
        child health collaboration
        research, 167, 172, 192
    funding of Minnesota birth outcome
        project, 87

Room to Grow
    building evaluation partnerships,
        115–20
    as center-based model, 135
    collaboration with Columbia
        University, 15, 111–12, 113–20,
        123–27, 133, 135, 139, 143, 205
    core values, 143
    data collection for, 118, 121–22, 133,
        134–40
    funding for, 120, 127
    as hybrid program model, 140
    impact of shelter system on, 126, 135–37
    interviews conducted for, 132–33, 136
    messaging and dissemination of
        research, 140–43
    services offered, 114–15
    social entrepreneurship in, 195
    study design and process evaluation,
        121–34
    team members, 111
    use of surveys in, 118, 127–29, 130,
        133–35, 139
    use of technology in, 121–26

Roots Community Birth Center
    as "best-practices clinic," 199
    early outputs, dissemination, and
        outcomes, 95–97
    establishes blog series, 84, 96, 101
    funding for, 87, 103, 106
    goals of, 84, 88–89, 92
    healthcare delivery system, 85–86
    history and goals of, 93–94
    mentorship, 102–3
    overview of program, 15
    racism and weathering as factors, 89–91
    single-payment reimbursement for, 106
    as site of research project, 92–93
    successes, 97
    team members, 83, 94–95, 205–6, 211
    time management, 104–5
    use of surveys for, 84, 125–26
    visibility and dialog in media, 98–99
    women's empowerment at, 99–100

Roselawn, Ohio, 14, 37, 40–42, 46–47, 49,
    51, 206, 209

S
segregation, 32, 85
    see also Roots Community Birth Center
self-care workshops, 158
Shaken Baby Syndrome, 169
Sister Friends (peer mentors), 26–27,
    29–30, 31–32
slavery, 32, 85
sleep duration and obesity, 151
smartphones, 153
smoking
    cessation policies in public housing, 37
    as risk factor in pregnancy, 90
SMS text service, 153
SNAP (food assistance), 126
social entrepreneurship for change, 194–95
Social Science and Medicine, 8
Social Services Appropriations (Utah), 178f
software, 74, 121
SPEAK UP Against Racism, 32
SPEAK UP for African American and
    Black Women, 32
spinal cord injuries, 37
stakeholders
    and at-risk infants, 176–83
    for Communities Acting for Kids
        Empowerment (CAKE), 36, 37,
        40, 42, 44, 46, 47, 49, 50, 51, 66
    in ICER projects, 200, 206
    need for diverse, 3
    for Puerto Rico WIC research, 149, 155,
        161–62
    for Room to Grow research, 143
    for Roots Community Birth Center, 84,
        92, 95, 96, 100
structural racism, 15, 85, 88, 93, 97, 99, 107,
    211

study cells, 138
stylus, 122
Su Casa Hispanic Center, 41
supermarkets, 157
surveys
    for CAKE research, 42, 44, 48
    on preschoolers and parental incarcera-
        tion, 57–58, 75
    for Puerto Rico WIC research, 153, 155,
        160
    for Room to Grow research, 118,
        127–29, 130, 133–35, 139
    for Roots Community Birth Center
        research, 84, 92
    web-based during postpartum period,
        84, 92
Svedin, Lina, 168, 171, 185–87, 189–90

T
tablets technology, 30, 31, 122, 126
taxes, 14
team building
    for Arkansas Birthing Project, 24
    importance of, 215
    for Indiana mass incarceration research,
        64–67, 69, 73, 197, 204, 210
technology.
    for Arkansas Birthing Project, 14,
        21–22, 24, 28–31, 33
    for Room to Grow research, 115,
        121–26
    for WIC program, 153
    see also specific technology
terminology
    differences in workplace, 72
    used by public health and academic
        medicine, 6
testifying (church tradition), 27
text messaging, 26, 71, 72, 95, 139
time management, 104–5

Topmiller, Michael, 35, 46
trauma
    Adverse Childhood Experiences
        (ACEs), 12
    healing from personal and historical, 15
Triple-P (Positive Parenting Program),
    131
turnover of caseworkers, 174, 181–82

U
Underground Railroad to New Life, 25
United States
    CBPR to improve health in, 8–11
    Census, 137
    child abuse and neglect in, 169–71
    childbirth care and outcomes in, 95
    childhood obesity in, 12, 150–51
    childhood poverty rate in, 41
    Congress, and authorization of PCORI,
        7
    funding for child welfare, 174
    funding for WIC program, 152, 155
    Health and Human Services Home
        Visiting Evidence of Effectiveness
        (HOMEVEE), 132
    history of segregation and racism in, 32
    legislation to support maternal
        mortality review, 101
    Maternal, Infant and Early Childhood
        Home Visiting (MIECHV), 131
    Medicaid funding, 93, 96
USDA-Food Nutrition Service, 155, 160
USPS, 139
University of Arkansas for Medical
    Sciences
    Center for Distance Health, 29
    Department of Obstetrics and
        Gynecology, 24
University of Puerto Rico, 154, 155, 157

University of Tennessee Health Science
    Center. Department of Health
    Promotion and Disease Prevention,
    25
Utah Children's Justice Center, 191
Utah child welfare and child health
    collaboration research
    barriers to collaboration, 172–76
    changes implemented, 200
    Child Fatality Review Committee, 178f
    Child Protection Ombudsman, 178f
    Child Welfare Improvement Council,
        178f
    Child Welfare Legislative Oversight
        Committee, 178
    community defined for, 177, 201–2
    and CPS, 167–73, 175–77, 179–82,
        185–86, 188–89, 192, 202
    Department of Human Services, Office
        of Services Review, 178f
    evaluation of research team, 197
    formation of team, 183–91
    funding for, 167, 172, 192
    importance of collaboration in, 205–6
    project goals, 16
    success of, 191–92
    team members, 167–69, 171, 204
Utah Division of Child and Family
    Services (DCFS)
    as community stakeholder, 176–82,
        178f, 189
    Myrup's role in, 171
    and pending legislation, 190
    as site for randomized controlled trial,
        172
    Svedin's participation in, 185

V
vocabulary differences, 3, 10

W
Waldfogel, Jane, 117, 120
weathering framework, 89–91
web sites
    American Journal of Managed Care, 96
    Arkansas Birthing Project, 27, 31, 32
    Birthing Project USA, 27
    for maternal mortality and morbidity,
        32
    for Puerto Rico WIC research, 153–56,
        158, 163
    University of Arkansas for Medical
        Sciences, 29
wellness, early childhood. *see*
        Communities Acting for Kids
        Empowerment (CAKE)
wellness model of pregnancy and birth. *see*
        Roots Community Birth Center

whites
    and access to health care, 88, 89
    and infant mortality rate, 87
    maternal age and birth weight, 90–91
    obesity rate among, 151
    and use of midwives, 86
WIC programs
    see Puerto Rico WIC research
Wi-Fi, 31
Wimer, Christopher, 111, 120
WomenVenture, 93
workplace culture, 72
wraparound supports, 141

Z
Zero to Three (nonprofit), 142